Patient Safety in Obstetrics and Gynecology

Editor

PAUL A. GLUCK

OBSTETRICS AND GYNECOLOGY CLINICS OF NORTH AMERICA

www.obgyn.theclinics.com

Consulting Editor
WILLIAM F. RAYBURN

June 2019 • Volume 46 • Number 2

ELSEVIER

1600 John F. Kennedy Boulevard • Suite 1800 • Philadelphia, Pennsylvania, 19103-2899

http://www.theclinics.com

OBSTETRICS AND GYNECOLOGY CLINICS OF NORTH AMERICA Volume 46, Number 2
June 2019 ISSN 0889-8545, ISBN-13: 978-0-323-67845-2

Editor: Kerry Holland
Developmental Editor: Kristen Helm

Obstetrics and Gynecology Clinics (ISSN 0889-8545) is published quarterly by Elsevier Inc., 360 Park Avenue South, New York, NY 10010-1710. Months of issue are March, June, September, and December. Periodicals postage paid at New York, NY, and additional mailing offices. Subscription price per year is $322.00 (US individuals), $685.00 (US institutions), $100.00 (US students), $404.00 (Canadian individuals), $865.00 (Canadian institutions), $225.00 (Canadian students), $459.00 (international individuals), $865.00 (international institutions), and $225.00 (international students). To receive student/resident rate, orders must be accompanied by name of affiliated institution, date of term, and the signature of program/residency coordinator on institution letterhead. Orders will be billed at individual rate until proof of status is received. Foreign air speed delivery is included in all *Clinics* subscription prices. All prices are subject to change without notice. POSTMASTER: Send address changes to *Obstetrics and Gynecology Clinics*, Elsevier Health Sciences Division, Subscription Customer Service, 3251 Riverport Lane, Maryland Heights, MO 63043. **Customer Service: Telephone: 1-800-654-2452 (U.S. and Canada); 314-447-8871 (outside U.S. and Canada). Fax: 314-447-8029. E-mail: journalscustomerservice-usa@elsevier.com (for print support); journalsonlinesupport-usa@elsevier.com (for online support).**

Reprints. For copies of 100 or more of articles in this publication, please contact the Commercial Reprints Department, Elsevier Inc., 360 Park Avenue South, New York, New York 10010-1710. Tel.: 212-633-3874; Fax: 212-633-3820; E-mail: reprints@elsevier.com.

Obstetrics and Gynecology Clinics of North America is also published in Spanish by McGraw-Hill Interamericana Editores S.A., P.O. Box 5-237, 06500, Mexico; in Portuguese by Reichmann and Affonso Editores, Rio de Janeiro, Brazil; and in Greek by Paschalidis Medical Publications, Athens, Greece.

Obstetrics and Gynecology Clinics of North America is covered in *MEDLINE/PubMed (Index Medicus), Excerpta Medica, Current Concepts/Clinical Medicine, Science Citation Index, BIOSIS, CINAHL, and ISI/BIOMED.*

Contributors

CONSULTING EDITOR

WILLIAM F. RAYBURN, MD, MBA
Associate Dean, Continuing Medical Education and Professional Development, Distinguished Professor and Emeritus Chair, Obstetrics and Gynecology, University of New Mexico School of Medicine, Albuquerque, New Mexico, USA

EDITOR

PAUL A. GLUCK, MD
Community Professor of Obstetrics and Gynecology, Florida International Wertheim College of Medicine, Miami, Florida, USA

AUTHORS

RAY ABINADER, MD
Fellow, Maternal Fetal Medicine, Eastern Virginia Medical School, Norfolk, Virginia, USA

MARISSA ABRAM, PhD, RN, PMHNP-BC
Board Chair, Pulse Center for Patient Safety Education & Advocacy, New York, USA; Assistant Professor, Adelphi University, College of Nursing and Public Health, Garden City, New York, USA

ARNOLD P. ADVINCULA, MD
Levine Family Professor of Women's Health, Vice-Chair, Department of Obstetrics and Gynecology, Chief of Gynecologic Specialty Surgery, Sloane Hospital for Women, Medical Director, Mary & Michael Jaharis Simulation Center, Columbia University Irving Medical Center, NewYork-Presbyterian Hospital, New York, New York, USA

SYLVIA AZIZ, MHA
MOC Program and Communications Manager, Maintenance of Certification, American Board of Obstetrics and Gynecology, Dallas, Texas, USA

CAITLIN BAPTISTE, MD
Fellow, Maternal Fetal Medicine, Department of Obstetrics and Gynecology, Columbia University Irving Medical Center, New York, New York, USA

BRIAN T. BATEMAN, MD, MSc
Chief, Division of Obstetric Anesthesia, Department of Anesthesiology, Brigham and Women's Hospital, Associate Professor, Harvard Medical School, Boston, Massachusetts, USA

DEBRA BINGHAM, DrPH, RN, FAAN
Executive Director, Institute for Perinatal Quality Improvement, Associate Professor, University of Maryland School of Nursing, Baltimore, Maryland, USA

DAVID J. BIRNBACH, MD, MPH
Miller Professor, Executive Vice Provost, Director, University of Miami–Jackson Memorial Hospital Center for Patient Safety, University of Miami Miller School of Medicine, Miami, Florida, USA

JASON BOULANGER, MFA
Program Director, Patient Safety, CRICO/RMF, Boston, Massachusetts, USA

ILENE CORINA
President, Pulse Center for Patient Safety Education & Advocacy, Wantagh, New York, USA

MARY E. D'ALTON, MD
Chair, Department of Obstetrics and Gynecology, Columbia University Irving Medical Center, New York, New York, USA

MARK S. DEFRANCESCO, MD, MBA
FACOG, Assistant Clinical Professor, Department of Obstetrics and Gynecology, University of Connecticut, Storrs, Connecticut, USA; Vice-Chair, Accreditation Association for Hospitals and Health Systems (AAHHS), Chief Medical Officer (Emeritus), Women's Health Connecticut, USA

ROXANE GARDNER, MD, MSHPEd, DSc
Assistant Professor, Obstetrics, Gynecology and Reproductive Biology, Harvard Medical School, Department of Obstetrics and Gynecology, Brigham and Women's Hospital, Division of Adolescent Gynecology, Boston Children's Hospital, Center for Medical Simulation, Boston, Massachusetts, USA

JONATHAN L. GLEASON, MD
Chief Quality Officer, Department of Clinical Advancement and Patient Safety, Carilion Clinic, Assistant Professor, Virginia Tech Carilion School of Medicine, Roanoke, Virginia, USA

DENA GOFFMAN, MD
Associate Professor, Department of Obstetrics and Gynecology, Columbia University Irving Medical Center, New York, New York, USA

DAVID HALPERIN, BA
Communications Director, Pulse Center for Patient Safety Education & Advocacy, New York, USA

ESTHER S. HAN, MD, MPH
Minimally Invasive Gynecologic Surgery Fellow, Division of Gynecologic Specialty Surgery, Department of Obstetrics and Gynecology, Columbia University Irving Medical Center, NewYork-Presbyterian Hospital, New York, New York, USA

ELIZABETH A. HOWELL, MD, MPP
Professor of Population Health Science & Policy and Obstetrics, Gynecology, and Reproductive Science, Director, Blavatnik Family Women's Health Research Institute, Icahn School of Medicine at Mount Sinai, New York, New York, USA

DAVID K. JONES, PhD
Assistant Professor, Department of Health Law, Policy and Management, Boston University School of Public Health, Boston, Massachusetts, USA

JOHN P. KEATS, MD, CPE, CPPS, FACOG, FACPE
Assistant Clinical Professor, Department of Obstetrics and Gynecology, David Geffen School of Medicine, University of California, Los Angeles, California, USA

CAROL KEOHANE, MS, BSN, RN
Assistant Vice President, Patient Safety, CRICO/RMF, Boston, Massachusetts, USA

WILMA LARSEN, MD
Associate Executive Director, Examinations, American Board of Obstetrics and Gynecology, Dallas, Texas, USA

ELLIOTT K. MAIN, MD
California Maternal Quality Care Collaborative, Clinical Professor, Department of Obstetrics and Gynecology, Stanford University School of Medicine, Stanford, California, USA

CATHIE MARKOW, RN, MBA
California Maternal Quality Care Collaborative, Division of Neonatal Medicine, Stanford University School of Medicine, Stanford, California, USA

DAVID MARX, BSE, JD
CEO, Outcome Engenuity

AMANDA NOVAK, MEd
MOC Program Administrator, Maintenance of Certification, American Board of Obstetrics and Gynecology, Dallas, Texas, USA

SUSAN RAMIN, MD
Associate Executive Director, Maintenance of Certification, American Board of Obstetrics and Gynecology, Dallas, Texas, USA

PAUL JAMES ARMAND RUITER, BMSc, MD, MCFP
Medical Director, Vice President, Salus Global, Knowledge Translation & Implementation Science Faculty, Canadian Patient Safety Institute, London, Ontario, Canada

STEPHANIE K. SARGENT, MHA, RN, CPPS (Certified Professional in Patient Safety), Certified Lean Six Sigma Black Belt
Vice President of Product Development and Quality, SE Healthcare, Charleston, South Carolina, USA

JEAN-JU SHEEN, MD
Assistant Professor, Department of Obstetrics and Gynecology, Columbia University Irving Medical Center, New York, New York, USA

POOJA SHIVRAJ, MS, PhD
Psychometrician, American Board of Obstetrics and Gynecology, Dallas, Texas, USA

ERIC SWISHER, MD
Assistant Professor, Virginia Tech Carilion School of Medicine, Roanoke, Virginia, USA

RICHARD WALDMAN, MD, FACOG
Chairman, Obstetrics and Gynecology, St. Joseph's Hospital Health Center, President, Associate for Women's Medicine, Syracuse, New York, USA

STEVEN L. WARSOF, MD
Professor of Maternal Fetal Medicine, Eastern Virginia Medical School, Norfolk, Virginia, USA

PATRICE M. WEISS, MD
Executive Vice President, Chief Medical Officer, Carilion Clinic, Professor, Virginia Tech
Carilion School of Medicine, Roanoke, Virginia, USA

ASHLEY YEATS, MD, FACEP
Vice President Healthcare Quality & Clinical Integration/Chief Medical Officer, Beth Israel
Deaconess Hospital–Milton, Milton, Massachusetts, USA

Contents

Focus on the Patient

Patient harm continues to be a leading cause of morbidity and mortality in the United States. Among high-risk industries, the health care system has a significantly lower safety profile than that of others. There are many driving forces behind this, including significant resistance within the medical community in the late 1960s to consumer demand of patient-centered and family-centered care. In subsequent decades the voice of the customer has taken center stage. The mounting research linking patient experience and engagement to patient safety and positive clinical outcomes is indisputable.

Keeping patients safe while they receive medical care is essential. Yet current systems designed to ensure patient safety are not enough, because medical error is the third leading cause of preventable deaths in the United States. Clinicians can partner with the patient to enhance patient safety. Pulse Center for Patient Safety proposes patient- and family-driven processes designed to improve a patient's chances of avoiding harm. This article discusses highlights of the role of patient safety through a grassroots lens, summarizes the factors that influence the patient's role in patient safety and reviews recommendations on how clinicians can partner with patients.

Preventable disparities in health outcomes for women during the perinatal period are unacceptable. To successfully combat these inequities, it is important to identify their causes and use quality improvement approaches to eliminate them. Proposed are 5 quality and safety strategies to guide efforts to eliminate disparities and ensure equitable health care for all women and newborns: (1) apply a systems approach based on the Socio-Ecological Model, (2) identify root causes of disparities, (3) identify and eliminate strong but wrong routines, (4) use improvement and implementation science methods and tools, and (5) use data to guide the plan and track progress.

Focus on Culture

Implementation and Change Management

Implementing change is difficult; few people want to wade into this area because of the challenge. However, it is highly rewarding and does not have to be complicated. Success requires a clear understanding of health care context, patient safety, and behavioral psychology. To achieve its goal, this article is divided into 3 parts: (1) the problem with engagement in health care, (2) patient safety in a new age, and (3) implementation.

Obstetrics and gynecology is a specialty practiced in some of the most complex care environments. Particular attention must constantly be paid to maintaining patient safety as a primary focus. A safe patient environment can only exist where leadership is committed to a patient-centric model of care delivery and creates a supportive culture. Safe patient care is best accomplished by teams. These teams need to understand and be committed to the concepts of open communication, situational awareness, and continuous learning.

Ensuring patient safety and optimizing outcomes in obstetrics and gynecology through improving technical skills, enhancing team performance, and decreasing medical errors has resulted in significant interest in incorporating drills and simulation into medical training, continuing education, and multidisciplinary team practice. Drills and simulations are ideal because of their wide range of application with various learners and settings. They provide a safe space to learn and maintain technical skills and to improve knowledge, confidence, communication, and teamwork behaviors, particularly for less common, high-stakes clinical scenarios.

Creating change at scale within a short time frame poses multiple challenges. Using the experience of the California Maternal Quality Care Collaborative, the authors illustrate how state perinatal quality collaboratives have been able to achieve this goal using a series of key steps: engage as many disciplines and partner organizations as possible; mobilize low-burden data to create a rapid-cycle data center to support the quality improvement efforts; provide up-to-date guidance for implementation using safety bundles and tool kits; and make available coaching and peer learning to support implementation through multihospital quality collaboratives. There are now multiple national resources available to support these efforts.

Emerging Clinical Trends

patient safety protocols. As various forces drove many surgical proced-ures to the ambulatory setting, many advantages, and perhaps several dis-advantages, quickly became apparent. In some studies, adverse events were found to be more common in office settings for instance, and it was quickly recognized that the formal quality controls that had evolved in the hospital setting were not always transferred to the outpatient facility. This article traces the development of health care's response to this challenge.

Conventional and robot-assisted laparoscopic gynecologic surgery offers many advantages over a traditional laparotomy. However, these minimally invasive approaches can present their own particular risks. To ensure pa-tient safety, procedures must be properly planned and performed by a skilled surgeon. Pre-operative patient optimization can help ensure safety and efficiency. Additional risks before starting the actual procedure arise from unique requirements for patient positioning and the need for perito-neal access. The authors discuss these risks and the importance of a thor-ough working knowledge of anatomy and surgical equipment (specifically conventional laparoscopic devices) to mitigate them.

OBSTETRICS AND GYNECOLOGY CLINICS

SERIES OF RELATED INTEREST

Clinics in Perinatology (www.perinatology.theclinics.com)
Pediatric Clinics of North America (www.pediatrics.theclinics.com)

THE CLINICS ARE AVAILABLE ONLINE!
Access your subscription at:
www.theclinics.com

Foreword

Patient Safety: Action Learning for Improving, Not Just Informing

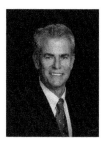

William F. Rayburn, MD, MBA
Consulting Editor

This issue of the *Obstetrics and Gynecology Clinics of North America* deals with patient safety in obstetrics and gynecology. It represents an update of the first issue on this topic in 2008 and is also capably edited by Paul Gluck, MD. While obstetrician-gynecologists have always striven to provide optimal care to their patients, health care has become increasingly complex, more dependent on technology, and reliant on teams. The issue is concisely organized into four sections: focus on the patient, focus on culture, implementation and change management, and emerging clinical trends. Articles in this issue are well referenced and shed new light on old problems while discussing emerging safety issues.

Efforts to improve quality and safety have achieved consensus as changes come from within departments. Transparency is critical for system improvement. Applying implementation science to the current concepts of patient safety will facilitate more rapid sustainable changes. Reliable data can identify opportunities for improvement and further encourage change by tracking progress.

Despite this, errors are always possible and under closer scrutiny by patients, the public, insurance companies, employers, and federal and local regulatory bodies. The patient safety movement has matured, and regulatory agencies are paying increasing attention to obstetrics and gynecologic care. Their critical role in advancing patient safety is now recognized. Patient satisfaction scores are directly related to reducing errors and improving outcomes. While many improvement efforts have been directed to the inpatient setting, the application of patient safety principles to outpatient settings is now gaining more attention.

I concur that "safety first" must be our mantra as new practices and technologies are introduced. The application of the patient safety techniques described in this issue is beginning to show improved care in a variety of women's health areas. More care is being delivered in ambulatory settings, and more minimally invasive procedures are

Obstet Gynecol Clin N Am 46 (2019) xiii–xiv
https://doi.org/10.1016/j.ogc.2019.02.003
0889-8545/19/© 2019 Published by Elsevier Inc.

performed in outpatient settings. Some results have more impact, less effort, less expense, and certainly less time in advancing care. This trend can result in greater efficiencies benefiting the patient, the provider, and the payer. Critical in this transition is recognizing the importance of safety, the value of teams, preparing for the unexpected, and effective, transparent communication.

Since the 2008 issue of the *Obstetrics and Gynecology Clinics of North America*, physicians have become more motivated to increase error reporting, identify hidden problems, and find and resolve system issues. In the wake of an error-related adverse event, great care is needed to avoid giving the obstetrician-gynecologist the sense that she or he is on trial for a crime or being targeted. Being human is not a fault. Otherwise, the potential exists of losing very capable doctors, if they either drop out or curtail their practice. At all times, physicians deserve maximal support as they meet the standard of care, incorporate lessons learned into practice, and commit to maintaining a relationship with the patient with full disclosure of events.

I appreciate Dr Gluck's effort to bring together leading advocates for improving patient safety in general, and in obstetrics and gynecology specifically, to increase our understanding and to suggest solutions. Expertise of the authors provides practical suggestions to reduce errors in the office, during surgery, and in labor and delivery. Their comments should provide a blueprint to continue advocating for safety in concert with medical innovation and personalized care.

William F. Rayburn, MD, MBA
Department of Obstetrics and Gynecology
University of New Mexico School of Medicine
MSC10 5580
1 University of New Mexico
Albuquerque, NM 87131-0001, USA

E-mail address:
wrayburn@salud.unm.edu

Preface

Patient Safety in Obstetrics and Gynecology: Some Progress, Many Challenges

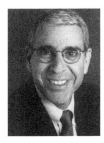

Paul A. Gluck, MD
Editor

Twenty years ago, the Institute of Medicine brought attention to the alarming number of patients harmed by medical care and suggested system level solutions. Since that time, we have made progress in addressing some issues. Other issues remain challenging, and new concerns have surfaced. Now new concepts have emerged with the potential to accelerate improvement. This issue sheds new light on old problems while discussing new safety issues.

The four aspects addressed by the contributors to this monograph are essential for lasting improvements in patient safety – patient engagement, culture change, implementation strategies and safety as a component in new healthcare trends.

Focus on the Patient (discussed by Waldman and Sargent; Corina and colleagues; Bingham and colleagues)

The critical role of the patient in advancing patient safety is now recognized. There is a rise of consumerism driving changes in medical care. Accelerated by links to reimbursement, patient satisfaction scores are directly related to reducing errors and improving clinical outcomes. Clinicians can effectively partner with patients and their families to significantly reduce medical errors and harm and improve patient satisfaction. Quality improvement methods can reduce disparities and improve health care for all populations.

Focus on Culture (discussed by Marx; Weiss and colleagues; Keohane and colleagues)

In order for any initiative to be implemented and sustained, there must be a receptive safety culture that is transparent and just and learns from mistakes. In a Just Culture,

Obstet Gynecol Clin N Am 46 (2019) xv–xvi
https://doi.org/10.1016/j.ogc.2019.02.002
0889-8545/19/© 2019 Published by Elsevier Inc.

obgyn.theclinics.com

unintentional slips result in changes to create a more resilient system. On the other hand, providers are held accountable for repeated and willful violations of accepted protocols. Transparency is critical for identification and analysis of errors resulting in system improvement. Patient Safety Organizations provide a mechanism for organizations to confidentially share common patient safety issues and learn from each other.

Implementation and Change Management (discussed by Ramin and colleagues; Ruiter; Keats; Goffman and Sheen; Markow and Main; Birnbach and Bateman)

The basic principles of patient safety are simple; implementation remains challenging. Approaching this problem from different perspectives may help accelerate and sustain change. The American Board of Obstetrics and Gynecology has integrated knowledge of patient safety into its initial as well as continuing certification processes. Applying implementation science to the current concepts of patient safety will facilitate sustainable change. Teamwork has long been recognized as important for the delivery of medical care in complex environments. Leadership, situational awareness, communication, and continuous learning are critical for well-functioning teams. Simulation has evolved from rudimentary models to high-fidelity environments. Ultimately, simulations have the promise of improving performance and patient safety. Reliable data can identify a need for improvement and then encourage change by tracking progress. Statewide collaboratives can use these data effectively to overcome barriers and to accelerate and sustain change.

Emerging Clinical Trends (discussed by Gardner; Baptiste and D'Alton; Abinader and Warsof; DeFrancesco; Han and Advincula)

Even though patient safety principles are universal, there are a number of emerging clinical areas where new strategies must be applied. These include a shift to more ambulatory care, procedures migrating from hospitals to outpatient settings, more procedures amenable to minimally invasive surgery, newer ultrasound technologies, and newer anesthesia techniques. Finally, an area that exemplifies how all these resources and strategies can be successfully applied concerns the need to reduce maternal mortality.

Reducing the number of patients harmed by well-intentioned but flawed medical care requires dissemination and implementation of proven best practices. In addition, new approaches are often necessary to solve old problems. "Safety First" must be our mantra as new technologies and practices are introduced. It is hoped that the expertise of the authors in this issue will provide a blueprint allowing patient safety to advance in concert with medical innovation.

Paul A. Gluck, MD
Florida International Wertheim College of Medicine
11200 SW 8th Street
Miami, Florida 33199, USA

1111 Crandon Boulevard
Suite A-308
Key Biscayne, FL 33149, USA

E-mail address:
pagluck@alum.mit.edu

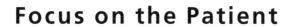

Focus on the Patient

The Patient Experience and Safety

Stephanie K. Sargent, MHA, RN, CPPS (Certified Professional in Patient Safety), Certified Lean Six Sigma Black Belt[a,*], Richard Waldman, MD[b,c]

KEYWORDS

- Patient safety • Patient experience • Patient engagement • Family-centered care
- Patient-centered care • Patient centeredness • Hospital Consumer Assessment of Healthcare Providers and Systems, Value-based purchasing

KEY POINTS

- Although early consumer-driven efforts in the 1960s to take more control of patients care experience was met with some opposition in the medical community, the patient experience has since taken center stage.
- Led by the Institute of Medicine, patient-centeredness has become a central foundation of health care quality.
- Research supports positive correlations between the patient experience and clinical outcomes.
- The patient experience will continue to be measured and reported by the Centers for Medicare & Medicaid Services for the foreseeable future, including value-based purchasing payment models.
- The future of the patient experience will be grounded in consumerism, transparency, and convenience.

HISTORY

The consumer and feminist movements in the United States in the late 1960s and early 1970s created an atmosphere of empowerment. Women began questioning all aspects of childbirth. Consumer tidal waves spread into the health care realm in that era and challenged traditional methods used in labor management that were not founded on scientific rigor. The dissatisfaction with twilight sleep, over-usage of narcotics for pain relief, rigid obstetricians and rigid hospital rules, and an environment that discouraged bonding and breastfeeding created a rebellion among young couples.

Disclosure Statement: R. Waldman: Quality Consulting Shareholder, SE Healthcare 151 Meeting Street Charleston, SC 29401. S. Sargent: Quality Consulting Vice President, Product Development and Quality, SE Healthcare 151 Meeting Street, Charleston, SC 29401.
[a] SE Healthcare, Charleston, SC, USA; [b] Obstetrics and Gynecology, St. Joseph's Hospital Health Center, Syracuse, NY, USA; [c] Associate for Women's Medicine, 935 James Street, Syracuse, NY 13203, USA
* Corresponding author. 926 Ashley Avenue, Charleston, SC 29403.
E-mail address: stephsarg2000@gmail.com

Encouraged by the writings of Grantly Dick-Read (Natural Childbirth in 1933; Childbirth without fear; the principles and practice of natural childbirth,1944), Doris and John Haire (The Cultural Warping of Childbirth, 1972), and Elisabeth Bing (Six Practical Lessons for an Easier Childbirth, 1967) and with the support of not-for-profit advocacy groups, such as the American Society for Psychoprophylaxis in Obstetrics (Lamaze) and the International Childbirth Association, couples attended childbirth classes to get the education that would allow them to have crucial conversations with their care providers. Armed with knowledge, they became advocates who challenged the status quo with their individual birth plans. Enemas, perineal shaves, isolated birthing, and heavy narcotic usage decreased. Fathers started attending vaginal births and cesarean sections. Babies were no longer separated from their mothers, and bonding and breastfeeding were encouraged. Hospitals and physicians initially were reluctant to adjust to these new practices; the medical establishment gradually adapted and ultimately joined nurse midwives to develop models of care they referred to as "family centered."

Family-centered care (FCC) required education, treated couples with dignity, respected couples' preferences, and allowed collaborations so that every birth was tailored to the needs and abilities of the birth setting, the providers, and the birthing couple in a safe environment. The key concept of FCC is that patients and families can make decisions about their health care if they are armed with knowledge and guided by professionals.

FCC is a partnership approach to health care decision making between the family and health care provider. FCC has been recognized by multiple medical societies, health care systems, state and federal legislative bodies, the Institute of Medicine, and Healthy People 2020[1] as integral to patient health, satisfaction, and health care quality. In 1992, the Institute of Patient and Family Centered Care established the 4 core concepts of FCC: dignity and respect, information sharing, participation, and collaboration. They attempted to define and enhance the concepts of FCC that had been so successful in the prior years in maternal and child care.

PATIENT CENTEREDNESS

Avedis Donabedian recognized that patient knowledge and satisfaction were important concepts in measuring quality.[2] Although Donabedian is referred to as the father of quality health care, he should also be regarded as the father of patient-centered care. The 2001 Institute of Medicine report, Crossing the Quality Chasm,[3] outlined 6 key aims for national health care quality improvement. One central aim was that health care be patient-centered; medical treatment should be "respectful of and responsive to individual patient preferences, needs, and values, and ensuring that patient values guide all clinical decisions."[3]

Hospital Consumer Assessment of Healthcare Providers and Systems

The patient experience measures are those most closely associated with patient engagement and optimal clinical outcomes. An example of a survey item in the Hospital Consumer Assessment of Healthcare Providers and Systems (HCAHPS) survey is, "When I left the hospital, I had a good understanding of the things I was responsible for in managing my health."[4] A patient who understands the plan of care is more highly engaged and could be more likely to adhere to recommended treatments and medications, leading to better health outcomes.[5,6]

HCAHPS is 1 of the Agency for Healthcare Research and Quality (AHRQ) family of CAHPS (Consumer Assessment of Healthcare Providers and Systems) surveys. Each evaluates a specific type of health care service. HCAHPS is a survey instrument and data collection methodology for measuring patients' perceptions of their hospital experience.[7] HCAHPS is driven by 3 goals[7]:

1. To establish objective and meaningful comparisons of hospitals on topics most important to consumers
2. To create new incentives for hospitals to improve quality of care by publicly reporting the data
3. To increase transparency and accountability by public reporting the quality of hospital care provided

HCAHPS was the first national, standardized, publicly reported information allowing consumers to make valid comparisons across hospitals. The development of the survey was the result of a partnership between Centers for Medicare & Medicaid Services (CMS) and AHRQ, both in the federal Department of Health and Human Services.

Rigorous testing of the survey instrument's validity began in 2002. The National Quality Forum (a national organization that represents the consensus of many health care providers, consumer groups, professional associations, purchasers, federal agencies, and research and quality organizations) endorsed the HCAHPS survey in 2005 and hospitals began using the HCAHPS survey voluntarily in 2006 for public reporting in 2008.

HCAHPS measures key aspects of care quality[8]: communication with nurses, communication with doctors, responsiveness of hospital staff, pain management, communication about medicines, discharge information, cleanliness and quietness of a hospital, overall rating of the hospital, and patient willingness to recommend the hospital. Because Medicare requires that hospitals collect and report HCAHPS data to receive their full annual payment update, HCAHPS quickly became the national standard for assessing patient experiences with hospital care.

HCAHPS data can be found at on the Hospital Compare Web site (https://www. medicare.gov/hospitalcompare/search.html?). The Web site posts the most current 4 consecutive quarters of data. To ensure fairness and accurate comparisons, factors that are not directly related to hospital performance but that affect how patients answer HCAHPS survey items are adjusted. Only the adjusted results are publicly reported.

Value-based Purchasing

With pay-for-performance programs beginning in 2009, CMS emphasized accountability. Today, the Patient Experience of Care Domain forms the basis for reimbursement in CMS value-based purchasing (VBP) programs, which introduced a model of health care organizations and providers reimbursement for the quality of care as opposed to solely basing payments on the volume of services (fee for service).

The name of the Patient Experience of Care Domain has evolved[9]:

- In fiscal year (FY) 2017 and (FY) 2018 it was called the Patient- and Caregiver-Centered Experience of Care/Care Coordination Domain
- In FY 2019 it will be called the Person and Community Engagement Domain

CMS makes incentive payments to hospitals based on either of the following:

- How well they perform on each of the 9 HCHAPS measures compared with other hospitals' performance during a baseline period
- How much they improve their performance on each measure compared with their performance during a baseline period

With the shift from fee for service to pay for performance, VBP effected an increased focus on improving the patient experience. Not only does improvement of patient experience scores increase reimbursement but also there are positive impacts on population health and clinical outcomes. For example, CMS does not reimburse for the incremental costs associated with health care–acquired infections.

MEDICAL COMMUNITY RESISTANCE
Controversy, Skepticism

Including patient experience as a pillar of safety and quality and treating patients in a humane and empathetic manner seem like common sense. Partnering with patients and listening to their concerns after thorough exchange of ideas is a superior way to practice that leads to a better patient experience.

Improving patient experience improves patient safety and effectiveness.[10–13] Providers have been slow to accept this concept. Critics became more vocal when reimbursements were tied to patient experience surveys. Many providers do not appreciate being judged by their patients and object to the survey methodologies. Providers frequently want proof that improving patient satisfaction improves safety.

Common criticisms of patient satisfaction survey include:
- Surveys are too long.
- Surveys do not adequately measure patient experience.
- There can be a significant delay in the time it takes for patients to fill out the surveys and surveys can be marred by recall bias.
- Surveys concentrate on superficial things, such as wait time.
- Only disgruntled patients fill out surveys.
- Survey data are not statistically valid.
- "They may not like the front office, but they like me."
- I cannot be judged adequately because there are too few responses.
- Slow feedback to providers who are in the trenches. Care was rendered months ago. By the time the reports are filtered through administrators the results are not operational.
- My patients are younger and, therefore, harder to please. Patients between ages 35 and 49 are simply harder to please. They want instant results.
- I am a woman and women rate lower on patient satisfaction scores with female patients.

Providers do not appreciate being judged by their patients:
- Patients are not qualified to judge us because they lack formal medical training.
- I did not become a physician to win a popularity contest.
- My patients are harder to please.

Academic objections:
- There are no randomized control studies that prove HCAHPS is related to safety or quality of care.
- Low scores do not translate to low-quality care. Patient satisfaction just isn't an objective measure of care quality.
- Minority patients may rate their visits as significantly less participatory than whites.
- Faced with penalties for low patient satisfaction scores, physicians could avoid caring for patients who may be more challenging to treat and perceived to be difficult to please, that is, underserved minorities, those with lower socioeconomic status and those with mental health concerns.
- Patient satisfaction surveys can call attention to the importance of treating patients with dignity and respect, but good ratings depend more on manipulability

and patient perceptions than on good medicine. In fact, the pressure to get good ratings can lead to bad medicine.

A common theme relates to situations in which good medically acceptable quality or value care is at odds with patients' understanding of good medical practice. The patient may desire antibiotics for their common head cold, for instance, yet the clinician will not provide antibiotics unless there is a clear indication. Denying patients antibiotics may be unpopular. Providers do not want to worry when they are advocating for good medical practices or when challenging patients with difficult conversations that their survey scores will suffer and their reimbursement might decrease.

THE SAFETY DATA

The Institute of Medicine defines patient safety as "...the prevention of harm to patients."[14] Robust patient safety programs emphasize systems of care delivery that (1) prevent errors, (2) learn from the errors that do occur, and (3) are built on a culture of safety that brings together a collaboration between health care professionals, organizations, and patients.

Until recent decades, traditional medical wisdom held a somewhat paternalistic model of health care delivery, where the physician was the sole source of authority. Patients rarely questioned physician-prescribed treatment plans. They were recipients of health care, not active participants. FCC in obstetrics and research demonstrating the association between the patient experience/engagement with positive clinical outcomes has increased the emphasis on the patient experience.

There are numerous studies that have explored the relationship between the patient experience and clinical outcomes, with varying results (although 1 study found it more common to find positive associations between the 2[15]). For example, higher patient satisfaction has been associated with better outcomes among those with acute myocardial infarction, congestive heart failure, and pneumonia.[16–18] The patient experience also has been associated with fewer complications[19,20] and adverse events[21] On the other hand, 1 large, national study showed that a better patient experience was associated with greater inpatient health care use, higher overall and prescription drug expenditures, and increased mortality.[22]

There are numerous other studies that support the impact of the patient experience on patient safety. Findings include the following:

- Patient experience positively correlates to processes of care for both prevention and disease management.[23]
- Patients' experiences with care, in particular communication with providers, correlate with adherence to medical advice and treatment plans.[24–27]
- Patients with better care experiences often have better health outcomes.[8,9]
- Good patient experience is associated with lower medical malpractice risk.[10,11]

Many health care organizations measure performance using pillars of defined business outcomes, such as growth, finance, quality, and people. The Institute of Medicine successfully advocated for the inclusion of patient experience as a measure by which to gauge quality.[28] Historically, the association between patient experience and clinical outcomes was less abundant. A metanalysis of 55 studies concluded that the patient experience has consistent and positive associations with patient safety and clinical effectiveness.[15]

Table 1 summarizes findings and presents the frequency of positive associations and no associations categorized by type of outcomes. These include objectively measured

Table 1
Associations with patient experience categorized by type of outcome

	Objective Health Outcomes	Self-reported Health and Well-being	Adherence to Treatment (including Medication)	Preventive Care	Healthcare Resource Use	Adverse Events	Technical Quality of Care	All Categories
No. of positive associations found	29	61	152	24	31	7	8	312
No associations	11	36	7	2	6	0	4	66

From Doyle C, Lennox L, Bell D. A systematic review of evidence on the links between patient experience and clinical safety and effectiveness. BMJ Open 2013;3:e001570; with permission.

health outcomes (ie, mortality, blood glucose levels, infections, and medical errors); self-reported health and well-being outcomes (ie, health status, functional ability, quality of life, and anxiety); adherence to recommended treatment and use of preventive care services likely to improve health outcomes (ie, medication compliance, adherence to treatment, and screening for a variety of conditions); outcomes related to health care resource use (ie, hospitalizations, hospital readmission, emergency department use, and primary care visits); errors or adverse events; and measures of the technical quality of care. The positive associations exceed those not found in every category reported.

Isaac and colleagues[29] demonstrate the relationship between the HCAHPS patient experience data and AHRQ patient safety indicators (PSIs) (**Tables 2** and **3**). PSIs are a set of 26 indicators providing safety-related adverse events occurring in hospitals after operations, procedures, and childbirth. PSIs are markers of hospital safety and quality. The study found statistically significant relationships between the patient experience and 2 medical PSIs: lower pressure ulcer and infections due to medical care. HCHAPS scores among the surgical PSIs showed statistical significance with pulmonary embolism or deep vein thrombosis as well as postoperative respiratory failure. Not surprisingly, among both the medical and surgical PSIs, the most consistent association was with "responsiveness of the medical staff." There was also a high correlation with "infections due to medical care" and "clean and quiet hospital environment."

A 2016 study sought to (1) document the association of PSIs and HCAHPS patient experience scores and (2) determine the risk-adjusted odds ratio of high patient experience scores compared with PSI presence.[30] The study found that 4.3% of patients had a documented PSI, the most frequent being hemorrhagic events (2.0%) and events related to obstetrics (1.5%). Obstetric-related PSIs include birth trauma rate–injury to neonate; obstetric trauma rate–vaginal delivery with instrument; and obstetric trauma rate–vaginal delivery without instrument). Risk-adjusted models showed patients with 1 or more PSIs had decreased odds of having high overall physician and nurse ratings. These results further support the relationship between the patient experience and quality of care (**Table 4**).

THE FUTURE OF THE PATIENT EXPERIENCE
Consumerism

The Internet has been a significant disruptor in health care and the patient experience. Online reviews are increasingly driving consumer decision making in the health care sector. Patients can easily discover a wealth of publicly posted information about health care providers. Web sites such as Healthgrades, WebMD, Physician Compare, Yelp, and Angie's List (to name a few), publish information on quality, safety, and patient ratings of health care providers.

Health care organizations are increasingly concerned with patient satisfaction–related measures, such as the comfort of a waiting room or amenity-laden birthing suites. These patient satisfaction–related measures can be associated with services, such as free Wi-Fi, coffee, or even providing individual desks or work areas with charging stations. Providing amenities such as these could prove beneficial as a satisfied patient is more likely to rate the provider higher and recommend the hospital or practice.

Consumers are approaching health care the same way they approach other consumer goods or services. Health care consumers are choosing providers with the highest patient experience ratings or the hospital with the highest safety measures (such as the lowest infection rates).

Health care consumers are more engaged. Although word of mouth and recommendations from friends and family continue to be influential, patients increasingly base

Table 2
Correlations between Hospital Consumer Assessment of Healthcare Providers and Systems ratings in medical service and medical patient safety indicators

Hospital Consumer Assessment of Healthcare Providers and Systems Rating by Medical Patients Measure	Medical Patient Safety Indicators					
	Decubitus Ulcer (n = 754)		Failure to Rescue (n = 755)		Selected Infection Due to Medical Care (n = 754)	
	Correlations	P value	Correlations	P value	Correlations	P value
Overall rating of hospital	−0.26	<0.001	−0.16	.20	−0.06	.38
Would recommend hospital	−0.28	<.0001	−0.22	.07	0.04	.53
Communication with doctors	−0.17	.005	−0.04	.76	−0.37	<.0001
Communication with nurses	−0.34	<.0001	−0.08	.55	−0.16	.01
Communication about medications	−0.26	<.0001	0.08	.60	−0.14	.07
Pain management	−0.24	<.0001	−0.14	.34	−0.07	.23
Clean and quiet hospital environment	−0.23	<.0001	−0.11	.38	−0.37	<.0001
Responsiveness of medical staff	−0.35	<.0001	−0.05	.71	−0.23	<.001
Discharge information	−0.22	<.001	−0.27	.05	0.08	.29

From Isaac T, Zaslavsky AM, Cleary PD, et al. The relationship between patients' perception of care and measures of hospital quality and safety. Health Serv Res 2010;45(4):1034; with permission.

Table 3

Correlations between Hospital Consumer Assessment of Healthcare Providers and Systems ratings in surgical service and surgical patient safety indicators

Hospital Consumer Assessment of Healthcare Providers and Systems Rating by surgical Patients Measure	Postoperative Patient Safety Indicators Complication Rates							
	Hemorrhage or Hematoma (n = 729)		Respiratory Failure (n = 711)		Pulmonary Embolism or Deep Venous Thrombosis (n=729)		Sepsis (n = 692)	
	Correlations	P value	Correlations	P value	Correlation	P value	Correlation	P value
Overall rating of hospital	0.17	.24	−0.33	.01	−0.03	.64	−0.08	.50
Would recommend hospital	**0.32**	**.03**	**−0.46**	**<.001**	0.004	.95	−0.16	.18
Communication with doctors	−0.11	.52	−0.30	.06	−0.07	.39	−0.19	.18
Communication with nurses	0.23	.14	**−0.36**	**.01**	−0.17	**.01**	0.12	.33
Communication about medications	NC[a]		−0.34	NC[a]	−0.20	**.01**	**−0.29**	**.05**
Pain management	0.23	.25	**−0.41**	**.006**	−0.15	**.04**	−0.09	NC[a]
Clean and quiet hospital environment	−0.11	.39	−0.14	.34	−0.09	.26	0.16	.18
Responsiveness of medical staff	0.08	.59	**−0.44**	**<.001**	**−0.21**	**.002**	−0.16	.19
Discharge information	−0.11	.50	0.24	.08	−0.18	**.01**	−0.27	**.04**

[a] Coefficient and P values were calculated using hierarchical model. NC indicates that the calculation did not converge due to insufficient data. Bold indicates statistically significant correlations (P<.05).

From Isaac T, Zaslavsky AM, Cleary PD, et al. The relationship between patients' perception of care and measures of hospital quality and safety. Health Serv Res 2010;45(4):1035; with permission.

Table 4
Adjusted odds ratios (95% CI) for having high overall physician and nurse experiences

Variable	Overall	Physician	Nurse
Patient safety indicators			
0	1.00	1.00	1.00
1 or more	0.86 (0.75–0.97)	0.76 (0.66–0.87)	0.83 (0.73–0.94)
Age (y)			
18–29	0.51 (0.45–0.57) 0.61	(0.53–0.70) 0.64	(0.56–0.72)
30–39	0.51 (0.45–0.57) 0.61	(0.53–0.69) 0.62	(0.55–0.70)
40–49	0.59 (0.52–0.67) 0.71	(0.62–0.80) 0.76	(0.67–0.86)
50–59	0.67 (0.60–0.75) 0.84	(0.75–0.95) 0.88	(0.79–0.99)
60–69	0.87 (0.78–0.97) 1.20	(1.07–1.36) 1.07	(0.95–1.19)
70–79	0.91 (0.81–1.02) 1.08	(0.96–1.22) 1.04	(0.93–1.17)
80 and older	1.00	1.00	1.00
Gender			
Male	1.01 (0.95–1.07)	0.86 (0.81–0.92)	1.07 (1.01–1.14)
Female	1.00	1.00	1.00
Marital status			
Single (never married)	0 99 (0.89–1.10)	1.01 (0.90–1.14)	0.93 (0.83–1.04)
Married/common law/living with partner	1.09 (1.02–1.17)	1.20 (1.11–1.30)	1.14 (1.06–1.22)
Divorced/separated/Widowed	1.00	1.00	1.00
Education level			
Elementary or junior high	1.75 (1.51–2.02)	1.52 (1.30–1.78)	1.33 (1.14–1.54)
Senior high (some or complete)	1.46 (1.28–1.66)	1.47 (1.28 to 1.69)	1.23 (1.08–1.41)
College/technical school (some or complete)	1.22 (1.08–1.39)	1.22 (1.07–1.41)	1.06 (0.93–1.21)
Undergraduate level (some or complete)	1.11 (0.97–1.27)	1.17 (1.01–1.35)	1.04 (0.91–1.20)
Postgraduate degree complete	1.00	1.00	1.00
Patient born in Canada			
Yes	0.84 (0.78–0.91)	0.89 (0.82–0.97)	0.97 (0.90–1.05)
No	1.00	1.00	1.00
Admission type			
Urgent	0.78 (0.73–0.83)	0.62 (0.58–0.66)	0.87 (0.82–0.93)
Elective	1.00	1.00	1.00
Most responsive provider service			
Family practitioner	1.18 (1.11–1.25)	1.09 (1.02–1.16)	1.09 (1.03–1.15)
Other	1.00	1.00	1.00
Discharge disposition			
Discharged home with/without support	1.34 (1.18–1.51)	1.30 (1.14–1.48)	1.16 (1.03–1.32)
Other	1.00	1.00	1.00
Charlson comorbidities			
0	1.00	1.00	1.00
1	0.96 (0.89–1.03)	0.90 (0.84–0.98)	0.92 (0.85–0.99)
2 or more	0.83 (0.75–0.97)	0.78 (0.66–0.87)	0.73 (0.65–0.80)

From Kemp KA, Santana MJ, Southern DA, et al. Association of inpatient hospital experience with patient safety indicators: a cross-sectional. Canadian study. BMJ Open 2016;6:e011242; with permission.

their chose of providers and hospital on information from the Internet. Prior to their visit, patients frequently have researched their medical condition, treatment alternatives, and preferred medications.

Since 2003, pharmaceutical industry spending on direct-to-consumer promotion in television, print (magazines and newspapers), radio, Internet, and other forms of mass media (billboards and direct mailings) has increased from $59 million to $1 billion.[31] Direct-to-consumer advertising for prescription drug products has both benefits and detriments to the consumer. Nonetheless, the impact on the patient experience could complicate clinical decision making for providers who find themselves in situations where patients request (or demand) medications or treatments not indicated for their condition.

Transparency

With the passing of the Patient Protection and Affordable Care Act in 2010 and the individual mandate to purchase health insurance, many patients selected high deductible health plans. With increased out-of-pocket expenses, consumers are focused on getting more value for their money. Thus, health plans and health care organizations are more transparent regarding cost as well as quality. Accustomed to shopping for good and services, patients want the most cost-effective care possible.

Health care organizations constantly monitor and try to improve their patient experience performance scores. They are concerned about the lasting impact of negative online reviews. The patient experience has become a key driver of a practice's reputation, profitability, patient volume, and ultimately success.

Convenience

As consumers have become more accustomed to health care as a commodity, the demand for convenience, including better access and communication, has increased.

Patient Web Portals

The use of Web portals where patients can message providers, enter and update personal health information, request appointments, check laboratory results, and request prescription refills has become increasingly common. Numerous studies have demonstrated that older adults are less likely to adopt portals even though they use the greatest proportion of health care resources.[32–34] This is expected to change as portals become more patient-centric. Overall adoption has increased year over year since 2012.[35] The future of patient portals will likely include more mobile-friendly applications, the dominant platform preference for consumers. Other projected advancements include:

- The organization and synthesis of multiple sources of health information, including disparate electronic health records and wearable devices data, such as fitness trackers
- Improved communication between providers and patients, such as reminding patients about their treatment protocols
- The ability for a virtual visit with a provider

Retail Health Care

There has also been a shift from the traditional model of private practice to new points of service. In-store clinics, such as those in CVS or Walgreens, debuted in 2000. They primarily treat minor infections and injuries and provide routine care, such as vaccination. These clinics increased 445% between 2006 and 2014.[36]

The American Medical Association has been a vocal critic of retail health care, citing concerns over quality and disrupting continuity of care between patients and the primary care physicians. A 2016 Rand research brief,[37] however, found that:

- Only approximately one-third of retail clinic users said that they had a primary care physician.
- Retail clinics offer quality of care comparable to that of physician offices and urgent care centers.

Retail models have found to be serving a population who do not otherwise have a relationship with a primary care physician and may otherwise seek care in an emergency department. Up to 20% of emergency department visits for a nonemergency condition could safely take place at a retail clinic or urgent care center, with an annual savings of $4.4 billion.[38]

The long-term impact of these care models on clinical outcomes and population health needs to be monitored.

Telemedicine

Beginning in the 1990s, telemedicine emerged as yet another consumer-driven method of health care delivery; 90% of health care executives have or will be developing a telemedicine program.[39] Telemedicine especially benefits the 20% of Americans who live in a rural area and have less access to care. From the patient experience perspective, however, all patients benefit. A systematic review explored the association of telehealth and patient satisfaction in regard to effectiveness and efficiency.[40] Factors relating to effectiveness and efficiency listed most often were improved outcomes (20%), preferred modality (10%), ease of use (9%), low cost (8%), improved communication (8%), and decreased travel time (7%).

Virtual visits both are convenient for patients and offer an efficient means for physicians to provide routine care for minor issues and manage chronic health conditions. Insurance companies are increasingly covering virtual visits. As organizations struggle to meet access demands and to perform well on patient experience measures, it is likely that telemedicine will increase.

Patient-reported Outcome Measures

Since 2009, The National Health Service in England has been measuring patient-reported outcome measures (PROMs). PROMs are subjective patient reporting on some elective surgical procedures. PROMs measure effectiveness and quality-of-life issues that go beyond HCAHPS surveys. They measure postsurgery health improvement from a patient's perspective. These data are publicly reported.

Similarly, the CMS Quality Payment Program (QPP) has implemented Meaningful Measures, moving toward outcomes-based measures and reducing the focus on process measures. PROMs include functional outcomes reporting, on procedures such as from orthopedic-related surgeries (eg, hip and knee replacements) to cataract surgery. To participate in QPP, a practice must submit data for at least 6 quality measures during a 12-month reporting period. Reflecting the impact of the patient experience on safety and quality, PROMs are given high priority within the QPP, and performance on PROMs has a direct impact on provider payments.

Reputation

Patients are increasingly using social media to post physician reviews online. Although online negative reviews seem to shape patient attitudes,[41] there seems to be no correlation between online physician ratings and outcomes, such as coronary bypass mortality rates among cardiovascular surgeons.[42] Online physician reviews do not correlate to formal institutional surveys, such as those by Press Ganey.[36] As a result, many providers are using third-party vendors to conduct their own patient experience surveys. They then display their star ratings to help market their practice.

SUMMARY

The effect of the patient experience on patient safety has been most impacted by ever-growing levels of patient engagement. Beginning with obstetrics and gynecology, patients have demanded patient-centered care and FCC and laid the foundation for the their application across all care settings.

With the rise of the Internet came myriad sources of information. Patients are increasingly educating themselves on their health-related conditions, treatment options, and alternatives. The Internet also provides a vast source of information on health care organizations quality and safety outcomes—data from regulatory agencies as well as social media sites. This has catapulted health care into a consumerism model, where patients are able to compare and shop for health care as they would any other commodity.

CMS and other regulatory agencies will continue to include the patient experience as a measure of quality and safety for the foreseeable future. Although the regulatory environment changes regularly, there nonetheless persists a focus on measuring the patient's perception of care. Recently, the additions of PROMs have been integrated into value-based reimbursement models.

There is a strong association between the patient experience, patient engagement, and clinical outcomes. This places the onus on the health care to develop innovative systems that use this information to empower patients and meet the objectives of Institute for Healthcare Improvement Triple Aim: improving the patient experience of care (including quality and satisfaction), improving the health of populations, and reducing the per capita cost of health care.

Organizations understand that addressing the patient experience is a business imperative. For organizations, engaged patients will improve safety, effectiveness, efficiency, and value. With an increasingly competitive environment and disrupted markets, organizations that embrace the patient experience will thrive.

REFERENCES

1. Kuo DZ, Houtrow AJ, Arango A, et al. Family-centered care: current applications and future directions in pediatric health care. Matern Child Health J 2012;16(2): 297–305.
2. Ayanian JZ, Markel H. Donabedian's lasting framework for health care quality. N Engl J Med 2016;375(3):205–7.
3. Institute of Medicine. Crossing the quality chasm: a new health system for the 21st century. Washington, DC: The National Academies Press; 2001.
4. Health Services Advisory Group. HCAHPS V13.0 Appendix A - mail survey materials (English) March 2018 materials. In: survey instruments. 2018. Available at: http://www.hcahpsonline.org/globalassets/hcahps/survey-instruments/mail/july-1-2018-and-forward-discharges/2018_survey-instruments_english_mail.pdf. Accessed September 23, 2018.
5. Vincent CA, Coulter A. Patient safety: what about the patient? Qual Saf Health Care 2002;11:76–80.

6. Coulter A. Engaging patients in healthcare. Maidenhead (United Kingdom): Open University Press; 2011.

7. Centers for Medicare & Medicaid Services. HCAHPS: patients' perspectives of care survey. In: HCAHPS overview. Available at: https://www.cms.gov/Medicare/Quality-Initiatives-Patient-Assessment-Instruments/HospitalQualityInits/HospitalHCAHPS.html. Accessed September 23, 2018.

8. Centers for Medicare & Medicaid Services. The HCAHPS survey – frequently asked questions. Available at: https://www.cms.gov/Medicare/Quality-Initiatives-Patient-Assessment-Instruments/HospitalQualityInits/Downloads/HospitalHCAHPS FactSheet201007.pdf. Accessed October 24, 2018.

9. Health Services Advisory Group. HCAHPS and hospital VBP. In: how CMS Calculates the Patient Experience of Care (HCAHPS) domain score in the hospital value-based purchasing program. Available at: http://www.hcahpsonline.org/globalassets/hcahps/vbp/hospital-vbp-domain-score-calculation-step-by-step-guide-february-2018.pdf. Accessed September 23, 2018.

10. Mehta SJ. Patient satisfaction reporting and its implications for patient care. AMA J Ethics 2015;17(7):616–21.

11. Boulding W, Glickman SW, Manary MP, et al. The patient experience and health outcomes. N Engl J Med 2013;368(3):201–3. Available at: nejm.org. Accessed October 23, 2018.

12. Nash IS. Why physicians hate "patient satisfaction": the real reasons. Ann Intern Med 2016;165(1):72.

13. Nash IS. Why physicians hate "patient satisfaction" but shouldn't. Ann Intern Med 2015;163(10):792–3.

14. National Academy of Sciences. Patient safety: achieving a new standard for care. In: Aspden P, Corrigan J, Wolcott J, et al, editors. Introduction. Washington, DC: National Academies Press; 2004. p. 29–44.

15. Doyle C, Lennox L, Bell D. A systematic review of evidence on the links between patient experience and clinical safety and effectiveness. BMJ Open 2013;3 [pii: e001570].

16. Glickman SW, Boulding W, Manary M, et al. Patient satisfaction and its relationship with clinical quality and inpatient mortality in acute myocardial infarction. Circ Cardiovasc Qual Outcomes 2010;3:188–95.

17. Jha AK, Orav EJ, Zheng J, et al. Patients' perception of hospital care in the United States. N Engl J Med 2008;359:1921–31.

18. Boulding W, Glickman SW, Manary MP, et al. Relationship between patient satisfaction with inpatient care and hospital readmission within 30 days. Am J Manag Care 2011;17:41–8.

19. Stein SM, Day M, Karia R, et al. Patients' perceptions of care are associated with quality of hospital care: a survey of 4605 hospitals. Am J Med Qual 2015;30:382–8.

20. Weissman JS, Lopez L, Schneider EC, et al. The association of hospital quality ratings and adverse events. Int J Qual Health Care 2014;24:129–35.

21. Black N, Varaganum M, Hutchings A. Relationship between patient experience (PREMs) and patient reported outcomes (PROMs) in elective surgery. BMJ Qual Saf 2014;23:534–42.

22. Fenton JJ, Jerant AF, Bertakis KD, et al. The cost of satisfaction: a national study of patient satisfaction, health care utilization, expenditures, and mortality. Arch Intern Med 2012;172:405–11.

23. Sequist TD, Schneider EC, Anastario M, et al. Quality monitoring of physicians: Linking patients' experiences of care to clinical quality and outcomes. J Gen Intern Med 2008;23(11):1784–90.
24. DiMatteo MR. Enhancing patient adherence to medical recommendations. JAMA 1994;271(1):79–83.
25. DiMatteo MR, Sherbourne CD, Hays RD, et al. Physicians' characteristics influence patients' adherence to medical treatment: results from the medical outcomes study. Health Psychol 1993;12(2):93–102.
26. Safran DG, Taira DA, Rogers WH, et al. Linking primary care performance to outcomes of care. J Fam Pract 1998;47(3):213–20.
27. Zolnierek KB, Dimatteo MR. Physician communication and patient adherence to treatment: a meta-analysis. Med Care 2009;47(8):826–34.
28. Institute of Medicine. A new health system for the 21st century. In: Crossing the quality chasm: a new health system for the 21st century. Washington, DC: National Academy Press; 2001. p. 23–38.
29. Isaac T, Zaslavsky AM, Cleary PD, et al. The relationship between patients' perception of care and measures of hospital quality and safety. Health Serv Res 2010;45:1024–40.
30. Kemp KA, Santana MJ, Southern DA, et al. Association of inpatient hospital experience with patient safety indicators: a cross-sectional, Canadian study. BMJ Open 2016;6:e011242.
31. Ventola CL. Direct-to-consumer pharmaceutical advertising: therapeutic or toxic? Pharm Ther 2011;36(10):669–74, 681-684.
32. Smith SG, O'Conor R, Aitken W, et al. Disparities in registration and use of an online patient portal among older adults: findings from the LitCog cohort. J Am Med Inform Assoc 2015;22(4):888–95.
33. Sarkar U, Karter AJ, Liu JY, et al. Social disparities in internet patient portal use in diabetes: evidence that the digital divide extends beyond access. J Am Med Inform Assoc 2011;18(3):318–21.
34. Graetz I, Gordon N, Fung V, et al. The digital divide and patient portals: internet access explained differences in patient portal use for secure messaging by age, race, and income. Med Care 2016;54(8):772–9.
35. Redelmeier DA, Kraus NC. Patterns in patient access and utilization of online medical records: analysis of MyChart. J Med Internet Res 2018;20(2):e43.
36. Accenture. US retail health clinics to double as focus shifts to clinical, including EHRs. In: View report: US retail health clinics expected to surge by 2017 according to Accenture analysis. 2015. Available at: https://www.accenture.com/t20160413T223640__w__/us-en/_acnmedia/Accenture/Conversion-Assets/DotCom/Documents/Global/PDF/Industries_18/Accenture-Chart-Retail-Health-Clinics-Double-by-2017.pdf.
37. Rand Corporation. The evolving role of retail clinics. In: research brief. 2016. Available at: https://www.rand.org/pubs/research_briefs/RB9491-2.html. Accessed September 23, 2018.
38. National Institutes of Health Health. How many emergency department visits could be managed at urgent care centers and retail clinics? Health Aff (Millwood) 2010;29(9):1630–6.
39. Foley, Lardner LLP. 2014 Telemedicine survey executive summary. In: download the 2014 telemedicine survey report. 2014. Available at: https://www.foley.com/2014-telemedicine-survey-executive-summary/. Accessed September 23, 2018.
40. Kruse CS, Krowski N, Rodriguez B, et al. Telehealth and patient satisfaction: a systematic review and narrative analysis. BMJ Open 2017;7:e016242.

41. Burkle CM, Keegan MT. Popularity of Internet physician rating sites and their apparent influence on patients' choices of physicians. BMC Health Serv Res 2015;15:416.

42. Okike K, Peter-Bibb TK, Xie KC, et al. Association between physician online rating and quality of care. J Med Internet Res 2016;18(12):e324.

The Patient's Role in Patient Safety

Ilene Corina[a,*], Marissa Abram, PhD, RN, PMHNP-BC,[b,1], David Halperin, BA[b,2]

KEYWORDS

- Patient safety • Partnering with patients • Patient's role in patient safety • Advocacy
- Health care bias

KEY POINTS

- Current patient safety protocols are not enough to prevent harm.
- A patient-, family-, and community-driven approach can be effective in improving patient safety.
- Clinicians can support techniques contributing to greater safety including communication, awareness of risks, hygiene, record keeping, medications, and respect. These techniques can be learned by patients and by their families.

Patient safety is at the heart of high quality health care. Without it, clinicians' best efforts and most advanced skills may be ineffective. In addition, the complexity of the health care and the human tendency for error can make achieving patient safety an ongoing challenge. Furthermore, the patient is a major stakeholder in the health care encounter influenced by diverse factors.

Health care is not as safe as it should be. It is estimated that 250,000 people die annually in the United States because of medical errors, making medical errors the third leading cause of preventable death.[1] According to a 2017 survey of more than 2500 adults, 21% reported that they personally experienced a medical error. When errors occurred, they had lasting impact on the patients' physical health, emotional health, financial wellbeing, or family relationships.[2]

Reports with estimates of death caused by medical error are somewhat controversial. Regardless, a serious medical error can have devastating impact on a family, causing a lifetime of emotional pain. This article will highlight the patient's role in patient safety and share recommendations on how clinicians can partner with patients.

Disclosure Statement: Authors have no commercial or financial conflicts of interest.
[a] Pulse Center for Patient Safety Education & Advocacy, P.O. Box 353, Wantagh, NY 11793-0353, USA; [b] Pulse Center for Patient Safety Education & Advocacy, Wantagh, NY, USA
[1] Present address: Adelphi University, College of Nursing and Public Health, One South Avenue, Garden City, NY 11530.
[2] Present address: 50 Glenwood Road, Roslyn Harbor, NY 11576.
* Corresponding author.
E-mail address: icorina@pulsecenterforpatientsafety.org

MEDICAL ERRORS

The report, "To Err is Human"[3] concluded that most medical errors do not result from carelessness or intent to do harm. Errors are caused by systems and processes that fail to catch and prevent human mistakes.[4] Medical errors are defined as "the failure of a planned action to be completed as intended or the use of a wrong plan to achieve an aim."[4] The outcome of this failure can result in harm to the patient. In health care, there are many opportunities for medical error, including miscommunication, rigid hierarchies, poor teamwork, medication administration, and prescribing.[5–7]

Although health care has become more effective, it has also become more complex, with new technologies, medicines and treatments. Health care organizations have been addressing patient safety by creating highly reliable processes. "Just Culture" (see David Marx's article, "Patient Safety and the Just Culture," in this issue) has created an environment that supports learning, designing safe systems, and managing behavioral choices to improve patient outcomes.[8–10] Patients often misunderstand the meaning of patient safety, equating it with health and wellness rather than the care that they receive.

THE PATIENT-FAMILY CONTRIBUTION

In 1996, Pulse Center for Patient Safety Education & Advocacy (Pulse CPSEA) began as a support group for survivors of medical errors. It was started by 3 parents (2 parents had lost a child, and 1 child had a child harmed by a medication overdose) who believed that they could improve safety by engaging the public. Patients and their families had important information often not considered in any root cause analysis of patients' injury or death. The first step in improving safety was discussing why errors happen. Pulse CPSEA has since grown into a community-based patient safety organization teaching advocacy and helping families.

Pulse CPSEA's educational work is based on stories—real experiences shared by real patients and their families. Almost any incident of a negative treatment outcome or bad health care experience can be mined for lessons. It is important to review how the medical error occurred and how it could have been prevented. Reflecting on strategies to address contributory factors such as communication issues is an essential first step that leads to solutions to prevent similar problems in the future.

CASE SCENARIO: SPEAKING UP

When Marlene, age 39, went into labor with her third child, a first-year resident administered an epidural that had been not been requested in the patient's birth plan. Prior to epidural placement her husband, Lenny, was asked to leave the room. He complied, feeling that the resident was a trustworthy authority figure. Lenny was not aware his wife would be receiving an epidural. Standing outside the room, Lenny heard his wife say, "Why does my head feel this way?" Concerned, he went back into the room. Immediately following the administration of the epidural, Marlene lost consciousness. She was declared brain dead a week later. Her heart stopped 19 days after the epidural, leaving her husband with 3 young children to raise without a mother. His oldest was 6 years old with severe disabilities and in need of round-the clock-care. Years later, the family still felt the devastation, especially Lenny, who sued the hospital and doctors to learn what happened. Lenny explained that if he had understood the risks related to epidurals he might have spoken up and stayed at his wife's side. He did not know that as a husband and the father his voice mattered. Marlene's death from medical error also affected her family, extended family, friends, and work associates.

Seeking transparency, accountability and system change, Lenny consulted an attorney who sued the physicians and the hospital. However, fewer than 10% of patients and families who experience a significant medical error file a malpractice suit.[11]

Family members or patients are often surprised when they cannot find a lawyer to take their case. The significant expense of malpractice litigation and contingency fees preclude many attorneys from pursuing malpractice cases even with obvious negligence. The average malpractice case costs $50,000 to litigate, with no guarantee the plaintiff attorney will be paid.[12]

If an attorney refuses a malpractice case, patients and families are left with questions and emotional suffering. If a case is settled, there is often a nondisclosure agreement precluding others from benefiting from the family's misfortune. It is important that patients and their families understand what happened when patients are harmed. Transparency, honesty, and apologies can restore trust and demonstrate that the needs of the patient and family are important. Furthermore, transparency is critical to inform system changes that will make medical care safer for everyone. Rather than condemning or penalizing the providers, understanding what caused the error may prevent reoccurrence. Concerns about malpractice hamper error disclosure. Error disclosure is uncomfortable. A recent patient safety primer reported that patients valued knowing that an error occurred, why it occurred, how the effects would be minimized, and what future steps would be taken to prevent reoccurrence.[13]

PATIENT AND CLINICIAN CONSIDERATIONS IN PATIENT SAFETY

Contributing factors for errors can be identified from the patient, the individual clinician, the organization, and the overall health care system. Patient safety in health care at the organizational level can be improved by creating highly reliable organizations with a just culture.[10–12] Patients can also be taught how to navigate the healthcare system in ways that will improve safety.

In a patient-centered approach the patient is an active participant in their health care facilitated by the clinician. This is essential for a culture of safety.

The clinician must actively engage patients for safety and patient satisfaction. Patient-related factors such as knowledge, belief systems, demographics, emotions, coping style, and the severity of illness can impact patients' willingness to actively participate in their care.[14–18] Patients usually believe that they are receiving competent care from an authoritative provider. Therefore, patients believe that their role is to follow instructions.[19] Perceived hierarchies can also act as an invisible barrier to patient participation.[20] Patients may fear speaking up because of concerns of offending the clinician or negatively affecting their care. Overall, patients want to listen, trust, and be cooperative.[21]

Clinicians can encourage and support active patient engagement. This can range from patients providing information that supports accurate diagnosis, to self-management, to monitoring treatment results. Although social determinants of health and varying levels of health literacy impact the patient-clinician interaction, ultimately the responsibility is shared, with the onus on the clinician. This in turn will result in improved compliance and better outcomes.

Promoting positive interactions between patients and clinicians offers opportunities to improve trust, increase understanding, improve outcomes, and remove blame in the event of harm from error. Even with well-intentioned clinicians, the health care environment can present challenges that include the lack of patient adherence and knowledge, poor communication within the health care team, time constraints, a desire to maintain the status quo, and fear of speaking up.[21,22] In addition, clinicians often do not recognize the significant risk of errors in health care, leading to complacency and failure to recognize errors in time to mitigate harm.

CASE SCENARIO: COMMUNICATION AND CLARITY

Lynette was distraught; she had received a call from her gastroenterologist's office stating that she had "spots on her uterus and kidney" and that she would need to follow up with her obstetrician/gynecologist and a urologist. While being evaluated by the obstetrician/gynecologist, Lynette complained of nonspecific abdominal pain. Concerned about a possible strangulated hernia, the obstetrician/gynecologist referred Lynette back to the gastroenterologist.

Lynette told the gastroenterologist that she felt the person who called from the office didn't explain the concern about the "spots." The doctor's body language changed; his demeanor went from friendly to tense. He reviewed the computed tomography (CT) scan and said, in a voice that seemed angry and impatient, that her CT scan was normal. Lynette's daughter, who was present, asked: "If this is normal, why did she have to be evaluated further?" This exchange was uncomfortable; the patient and her daughter could see that the doctor was annoyed, so they maintained a passive role. They felt intimidated, and their trust and confidence in the doctor was broken.

The Joint Commission reported that from 2011 to 2013, the most common root causes of a sentinel event were a communication breakdowns.[23] In Lynette's case, communication breakdown negatively impacted both the patient and the clinician. What could have been done differently? How could Lynette's distress (and financial cost) have been reduced? How could the doctor have felt less defensive? By communicating accurately and clearly on one hand and a patient empowered to ask clarifying questions on the other. It's about establishing a true partnership between the physician (and the physician's staff), the patient, and the patient's family.

BASIC RECOMMENDATIONS FOR PARTNERING WITH PATIENTS

One of the Joint Commission's national patient safety goals required health care organizations to "encourage patients' active involvement in their own care as a patient safety strategy." This goal catalyzed research on how patients may partner with providers to prevent errors and how patients may themselves inadvertently precipitate errors. Safer health care requires a collaborative effort by the public and medical professionals. There are a few ways that everyone can work together to improve patient safety.

Educate Patients to Be Aware of Risks

Patients need to be fully aware of the risks of care. Patients who engage in health care decisions with their provider "are less likely to regret their choices they make and more likely to comply with the treatment regimens they select."[23]

Encourage Patients to Keep Accurate Records

Patients can also provide key information that will improve the quality of their care by keeping an accurate and current medical history.[19]

Choose a Health Care Advocate

Patients should be encouraged to bring someone with them to collect and share important health care information. This person should understand his or her support role before interacting with the clinician. Because family members are emotionally involved, they may not always be the best advocates. Choosing the right advocate is important for receiving the best care. A family member advocate who dominates the discussion or has limited understanding of the health care system may cause more problems. In circumstances in which family members may become too emotional, such as a diagnosis of cancer, a friend or neighbor may be a more objective advocate.

The advocate might take notes during visits; ask the doctor questions; check medications; and in the hospital, verify details of a treatment plan, help reduce the risks of falls, guide food choices, ensure sanitary practices are followed, and question potential risks to the patient's well-being.

SPECIAL ISSUES IN PATIENT SAFETY

Certain issues are critical to the success of any patient safety improvement effort. Some, such as effective communication, are basic working principles while others, such as opioid use, are determined by circumstances.

Special Issue: Documents

Patients should be encouraged to name a health care proxy in advance: a person legally appointed by the patient to make health care decisions when they are unable. This role should not be confused with that of an advocate who helps when the patient can speak for him- or herself.

Special Issues: Opioids and Medication Management

According to the National Institute on Drug Abuse, every day more than 115 people in the United States die from opioid overdose.[24]

Twenty-one percent to 29% of individuals prescribed opioids for chronic pain misuse them.[25] If opioids are prescribed, health care professionals must explain the addictive potential to the patient. Similarly, postoperative patients must understand the addictive potential of many analgesics.

Noncompliance and misuse of many medications by patients, whether intentional or accidental, is widespread.[26–28] Clinicians can mitigate adherence issues by clearly communicating the risks of non-adherence and supporting the patient in developing self-management skills.[29]

Self-management is defined as "the ability of the individual, in conjugation with family, community, and health professionals, to manage symptoms, treatments, lifestyle changes, and psychosocial, cultural, and spiritual consequences of chronic disease."[30]

Nonadherence can be exacerbated by cognitive impairment caused by age, medication, or mental illness.[31–33] Pulse CPSEA recommends that every patient at risk for cognitive impairment, as well as minors, choose a designated medication manager (DMM) to help ensure that medications are taken (and stored) correctly. The DMM should also prepare and keep a list of all current medications.

Special Issues: Diagnosis

Diagnostic errors can occur when patients do not give a complete and accurate description of their symptoms. At Pulse CPSEA, adults and students are taught how to accurately describe their symptoms. They learn to describe what they were doing before their pain started, what improves the pain, whether there are any associated symptoms, and the severity of the pain on a scale of 1 to 10. Using roleplay, students learn that saying "I don't feel good" will not help to make an accurate diagnosis.

Special Issues: Health Literacy

In all conversations involving patients, providers, advocates, and families clear, courteous, and respectful communication in a nonthreatening environment is essential. However, it needs to be balanced by a firm but diplomatic readiness by the patient or their advocate to challenge practices or decisions perceived to be dangerous, inappropriate, or outside the agreed treatment plan. Patients and those supporting them must learn to speak up. Clinicians should also be aware that the patient might not fully understand the diagnosis or recommended treatment. Using validated tools, such as teach back, the provider should confirm the patient's understanding. Additionally, the patient should feel empowered to raise any concerns or request further explanations.

TOOLS FOR CLINICIANS

Patients should be encouraged to ask questions. There are numerous tools to support clinician - patient communication. The Agency for Healthcare Research and Quality's (AHRQ) Questions Are the Answer[34] program and 20 Tips to Help Prevent Medical Errors[33] fact sheet, as well as The Joint Commission's Speak Up[35] initiative help educate patients about safety hazards by providing them with specific questions. The Institutes of Healthcare Improvement (IHI) Ask Me 3 suggests important questions to be answered in each health care interaction: What is my main problem? (the diagnosis); What do I need to do? (treatment); and Why is it important for me to do this? (improve compliance).[36] For example, instead of saying "hypertension," clinicians should say "your main problem is high blood pressure." For treatment, instead of saying "sodium restriction," say "limit the amount of salt you add and avoid food that that contains a lot of salt." To create value for the treatment, the clinician can say, "The reason you need to reduce the amount of salt in your food and take your high blood pressure medications is that untreated high blood pressure can cause serious damage to heart and kidneys. It can increase the risk for strokes. Patients with uncontrolled high blood pressure may die prematurely." Patient engagement can be encouraged with posters and brochures from IHI and AHRQ.

At Pulse CPSEA, the A.S.K. for Your Life and Think S.T.A.R.S. principles are taught to community participants as ways to become more involved in their care. ASK for Your Life encourages patients to keep asking questions until they understand the clinician, and to speak up if they have any concerns (**Table 1**). Using the Think STARS method, participants take turns practicing describing their symptoms. STARS has been offered in high school classes and at community meetings about patient safety. All of participants in the training sessions reported that they felt better prepared to share information with their clinician.

THE TEACH BACK METHOD

The Teach Back Method is a tool with which the clinician confirms that patients understand and knows how to manage their health.[37] This can be done by asking patients to explain what the clinician taught them. The clinician can then clarify any misunderstandings. This has been shown to improve adherence and self-efficacy.[38] It is an important tool to maximize patient understanding and to promote self-management. Although teach back is particularly valuable for vulnerable groups,

Table 1		
Acronyms to teach patients about partnering in their care		
Ask Me 3	A.S.K. for Your Life	Think S.T.A.R.S.
1. What is my main problem?	Ask questions until you understand answers.	Specifics- specific location and/or what you were doing before it started
2. What do I need to do?	Speak up if something is not right.	Treatment-Are you taking medication, are you on a new medication, do you know the names and doses or your medication? Are you treating the pain with heat or cold?
3. Why is this important for me to do?	Know your body, your conditions, your medications and test results.	Associated symptoms-Are you experiencing dizziness, racing heart, bleed, nausea, or vomiting?
		Relieve or provoke the symptoms-What makes it feel better or worse?
		Severity- On a scale of 1–10, 10 being the worst, how are you affected?

such as African-Americans, the elderly, and less educated and non-English speakers, many other patients might also benefit from this method.[39]

AN INNOVATIVE COMMUNITY RESOURCE

There are many challenges in educating patients about patient safety including time constraints, the patient's emotional state, and individualized treatment plans.[40,41] One approach to help overcome these barriers is community patient safety education programs such as Pulse CPSEA. Pulse CPSEA focuses on teaching community members about safe, quality health care practices so they may become "knowledgeable, confident, and active participants in their healthcare experience." Pulse CPSEA also "provides a platform for effective communication and working partnerships whereby the community works with healthcare providers and institutions to proactively contribute to, and advocate for, safe quality care." Through mechanisms such as focus groups and stories of patient experiences, Pulse CPSEA actively listens to learn. This information is then utilized to develop programs partnering with local and national patient safety leaders to close the identified gaps.[42] This especially helpful when caring for vulnerable populations such as those with low English proficiency, people with mental illness or a disease with stigma such as human immunodeficiency virus (HIV)/ acquired immunodeficiency syndrome (AIDS).

FAMILY-CENTERED PATIENT ADVOCATE TRAINING

The Pulse Family-Centered Patient Advocate Training is an 8-hour program during which participants learn about patient safety and advocacy. Topics include preventing falls, avoiding infections and medication errors, and improving communication. As the public learns about patient safety they also learn how errors happen and how they can help to avoid them. In a recent course there was a 50% improvement in patient safety knowledge from the pretest to the post-test scores. After completing the program, participants are encouraged to volunteer as patient advocates.

PATIENT ACTIVATION THROUGH COMMUNITY CONVERSATIONS

Patient Activation through Community Conversations (PACC) are small group discussions with patients. These can be for individuals with a similar diagnosis such as cancer or people who are part of a vulnerable patient population such as limited English proficiency, the homeless, transgender people, or teen mothers. The PACC discussions help participants learn from each other to improve health care outcomes. The PACC starts with 50 questions on topics from which participants choose. Each question is meant to start a discussion, such as "Do you keep a list of medications at all times, and if so, do you include vitamins?" or "Have you ever changed doctors, and if so how, did you find a new one?"

When everyone has marked what they want to talk about, they pass their list to the facilitator. Then the facilitator reads what was checked off to begin the discussion. A strict rule is that there is no asking of questions. If someone said he or she did not understand their medical diagnosis, no one may ask what the diagnosis was or what the doctor said. If a participant wants recommendations, participants can speak only out of their lived experience. This might be responding to someone who wants to discuss how to choose a hospital. Participants are not to say, "This is what you should do…." Instead they might say "When I chose a hospital I asked my neighbors about their experience." Participants can only share what worked for them. This helps to avoid negativity.

A.S.K. FOR YOUR LIFE CAMPAIGN: ADDRESSING RACIAL BIAS

Nationally, the maternal death rate is 3 to 4 times higher among black women compared with white women.[43] In some communities, such as New York City, this disparity is even greater, with up to a 12-fold increase in maternal deaths among black women. Despite many calls by the medical establishment to address these disparities, the gap between the death rates of black women and white women from pregnancy complications is growing wider (See Debra Bingham and colleagues' article, "Quality Improvement Approach to Eliminate Disparities in Perinatal Morbidity and Mortality," in this issue).[44] Pulse CPSEA developed the A.S.K. For Your Life Campaign to address this issue. This initiative is spearheaded by an African American team consisting of a nurse and a retired obstetrician/gynecologist. The focus is on empowering the black community to recognize and deal with racial bias in order obtain safer health care.

It is a multimedia, interactive educational program with techniques and communication skills recommended by experts in patient safety and health care disparities.[45]

Most participants who completed the program say that they are asking more questions, speaking up if something's not right, and claim they experience less fear or intimidation during their encounters with clinicians.

OTHER VULNERABLE POPULATIONS

There are other populations at risk for discrimination and bias including transgender people, teenage mothers, HIV-positive patients, immigrants, homosexuals, and lesbians. Immigrant workers are especially vulnerable by virtue of language, poverty, lack of education, and sometimes residence status. Beginning in 2015, over an 18-month period, experts from Pulse CPSEA made weekly visits to a trailer on Long Island where day laborers meet to take classes and get work. Fifty-five Spanish-speaking people participated in the 18-month patient safety education course designed to improve health literacy. Low health literacy is generally associated with health inequalities, poorer health, a greater risk of hospitalization, and more costly care.[46–48] The project achieved its intended goal with a measurable change in behavior regarding health care.

Typical comments include

- Learned the importance of following instructions with any medication
- Learned how to ask questions regarding medications

- Learned the importance of asking for an interpreter
- Learned to ask the doctor about health conditions, and to ask questions if they did not understand
- Helped to be more assertive

SUMMARY

Families can also be taught to be more involved in patient safety. When one compares health care safety practices with those of airline industry, there are clear lessons.

In 2009, a bird strike caused the emergency landing of a plane on the Hudson River in New York. Captain Chesley Burnett Sullenberger III and the flight crew are credited with saving the lives of the passengers by safely ushering them out of the plane.[49]

But there is another side to the story. Before any flight takes off, airline passengers are told what to do in an emergency. Those of us who fly often can probably repeat these instructions from memory. Flight 1549's passengers were prepared and were part of the reason for a safe evacuation.

If they are taught how, patients and their families can also be part of the process, keeping themselves safe and avoiding medical injury. When educated, patients become a valuable resource. Through their engagement they can help prevent errors from happening, or if an error does occur, they can help prevent harm. Health care professionals should welcome and encourage active participation of patients and their families.

REFERENCES

1. Makary MA, Daniel M. Medical error—the third leading cause of death in the US. BMJ 2016;353:i2139. Available at: https://www.bmj.com/content/353/bmj.i2139.
2. Available at: http://www.ihi.org/about/news/Documents/IHIPressRelease_Patient_Safety_Survey_Sept28_17.pdf. Accessed February 3, 2018.
3. Kohn LT, Corrigan J, Donaldson MS. To err is human: building a safer health system. Washington, DC: National Academy Press; 2000. Available at: http://www.nationalacademies.org/hmd/~/media/Files/Report%20Files/1999/To-Err-is-Human/To%20Err%20is%20Human%201999%20%20report%20brief.pdf.
4. Agency for Healthcare Research and Quality. 2017. Available at: https://psnet.ahrq.gov/primers/primer/21. Accessed May 5, 2018.
5. Aronson JK. Medication errors: definitions and classification. Br J Clin Pharmacol 2009;67(6):599–604.
6. Freischlag JA, Holzmueller CG, Pronovost PJ, et al. Operating room teamwork among physicians and nurses: teamwork in the eye of the beholder. J Am Coll Surg 2006;202:746–52.
7. Taran S. An examination of the factors contributing to poor communication outside the physician-patient sphere. Mcgill J Med 2011;13(1):86.
8. Pronovost PJ, Berenholtz SM, Goeschel CA, et al. Creating high reliability in health care organizations. Health Serv Res 2006;41(4 Pt 2):1599–617.
9. Boysen PG. Just culture: a foundation for balanced accountability and patient safety. Ochsner J 2013;13(3):400–6.
10. Marx, DA. Patient safety and the "just culture": a primer for health care executives. Trustees of Columbia University. Available at: https://www.chpso.org/sites/main/files/file-attachments/marx_primer.pdf. Accessed February 3, 2018.
11. Medscape. Available at: https://www.medscape.com/viewarticle/814876_2. (Registration required). Accessed April 2, 2018.

12. Medscape. Available at: https://www.medscape.com/viewarticle/814876_2. (Registration required). Accessed April 2, 2018.

13. Agency for Healthcare Research and Quality. Disclosure of errors. 2018. Available at: https://psnet.ahrq.gov/primers/primer/2/disclosure-of-errors. Accessed April 2, 2018.

14. Davis RE, Jacklin R, Sevdalis N, et al. Patient involvement in patient safety: what factors influence patient participation and engagement? Health Expect 2007; 10(3):259–67.

15. Longtin Y, Sax H, Leape LL, et al. Patient participation: current knowledge and applicability to patient safety. Mayo Clin Proc 2010;85(1):53–62.

16. Lyons Melinda M. Should patients have a role in patient safety? A safety engineering view. Qual Saf Health Care 2007;16:140–2. Available at: https://www.ncbi. nlm.nih.gov/pmc/articles/PMC2653153/pdf/140.pdf.

17. Severinsson IE, Holm AL. Patients' role in their own safety—a systematic review of patient involvement in safety. Open Journal of Nursing 2015;(3):642–53.

18. Rainey H, Ehrich K, Mackintosh N, et al. The role of patients and their relatives in 'speaking up'about their own safety–a qualitative study of acute illness. Health Expect 2015;18(3):392–405.

19. Rathert C, Huddleston N, Pak Y. Acute care patients discuss the patient role in patient safety. Health Care Manage Rev 2011;36(2):134–44.

20. Langer T, Martinez W, Browning DM, et al. Patients and families as teachers: a mixed methods assessment of a collaborative learning model for medical error disclosure and prevention. BMJ Qual Saf 2016;25(8):615–25.

21. Okuyama A, Wagner C, Bijnen B. Speaking up for patient safety by hospital-based health care professionals: a literature review. BMC Health Serv Res 2014;14(1):61.

22. Hanson HM, Warkentin L, Wilson R, et al. Facilitators and barriers of change toward an elder-friendly surgical environment: perspectives of clinician stakeholder groups. BMC Health Serv Res 2017;17(1):596.

23. Advisory Board. Available at: https://www.advisory.com/daily-briefing/2017/03/01/get-patients-involved. Accessed March 1, 2017.

24. Davis RE, Jacklin R, Sevdalis N, et al. Opioid overdose crisis. NIH National Institute on Drug Abuse; 2018. Available at: https://onlinelibrary.wiley.com/doi/full/10.1111/j.1369-7625.2007.00450.x. Accessed March 14, 2018.

25. Vowles KE, McEntee ML, Julnes PS, et al. Rates of opioid misuse, abuse, and addiction in chronic pain: a systematic review and data synthesis. Pain 2015; 156(4):569–76.

26. Bosworth HB, Granger BB, Mendys P, et al. Medication adherence: a call for action. Am Heart J 2011;162(3):412–24.

27. Markotic F, Vrdoljak D, Puljiz M, et al. Risk perception about medication sharing among patients: a focus group qualitative study on borrowing and lending of prescription analgesics. J Pain Res 2017;10:365.

28. Vrijens B, Antoniou S, Burnier M, et al. Current situation of medication adherence in hypertension. Front Pharmacol 2017;8:100.

29. Costa E, Giardini A, Savin M, et al. Interventional tools to improve medication adherence: review of literature. Patient Prefer Adherence 2015;9:1303.

30. Wilkinson A, Whitehead L. Evolution of the concept of self-care and implications for nurse: a literature review. Int J Nurs Stud 2009;46:1143–7.

31. Fischer MA, Jones JB, Wright E, et al. A randomized telephone intervention trial to reduce primary medication nonadherence. J Manag Care Spec Pharm 2015; 21(2):124–31.

32. Velligan DI, Sajatovic M, Hatch A, et al. Why do psychiatric patients stop antipsychotic medication? A systematic review of reasons for nonadherence to medication in patients with serious mental illness. Patient Prefer Adherence 2017;11:449.
33. Available at: https://www.ahrq.gov/patients-consumers/care-planning/errors/20tips/index.html. Accessed April 2, 2018.
34. Available at: https://www.ahrq.gov/topics/questions-are-answer.html. Accessed April 2, 2018.
35. Available at: https://www.jointcommission.org/speakup.aspx. Accessed April 2, 2018.
36. Institute for Healthcare Improvement. In: Tools. Ask me 3: good questions for your good health. Available at: http://www.ihi.org/resources/Pages/Tools/Ask-Me-3-Good-Questions-for-Your-Good-Health.aspx. Accessed April 2, 2018.
37. Health literacy universal precautions toolkit. 2nd edition. Use the Teach-Back Method: Tool #5. Available at: https://www.ahrq.gov/professionals/quality-patient-safety/quality-resources/tools/literacy-toolkit/healthlittoolkit2-tool5.html. Accessed April 2, 2018.
38. White M, Garbez R, Carroll M, et al. Is "teach-back" associated with knowledge retention and hospital readmission in hospitalized heart failure patients? J Cardiovasc Nurs 2013;28(2):137–46.
39. Jager AJ, Wynia MK. Who gets a teach-back? Patient-reported incidence of experiencing a teach-back. J Health Commun 2012;17(3):294–302.
40. Gay C, Chabaud A, Guilley E, et al. Educating patients about the benefits of physical activity and exercise for their hip and knee osteoarthritis. Systematic literature review. Ann Phys Rehabil Med 2016;59(3):174–83.
41. McGinty EE, Thompson DA, Pronovost PJ, et al. Patient, provider, and system factors contributing to patient safety events during medical and surgical hospitalizations for persons with serious mental illness. J Nerv Ment Dis 2017;205(6):495.
42. Pulse Center for Patient Safety Education & Advocacy. About us. Available at: https://pulsecenterforpatientsafety.org/about-us/. Accessed June 9, 2018.
43. Agency for Healthcare Research and Quality. Healthcare cost and utilization project: statistical brief #222 delivery hospitalizations involving preeclampsia and eclampsia, 2005–2014. Available at: https://www.hcup-us.ahrq.gov/reports/statbriefs/sb222-Preeclampsia-Eclampsia-Delivery-Trends.pdf. Accessed June 9, 2018.
44. Lu MC, Kotelchuck M, HoganV JL, et al. Closing the black-white gap in birth outcomes: a life-course approach. Ethn Dis 2010;20(1 Suupl 2). S2–62-76.
45. Pulse Center for Patient Safety Education & Advocacy. Ask for your life campaign. Available at: http://askforyourlife.com/about-us/. Accessed June 9, 2018.
46. Smith SG, O'Conor R, Curtis LM, et al. Low health literacy predicts decline in physical function among older adults: findings from the LitCog cohort study. J Epidemiol Community Health 2015;69(5):474–80.
47. Boyle J, Speroff T, Worley K, et al. Low health literacy is associated with increased transitional care needs in hospitalized patients. J Hosp Med 2017;12(11):918–24.
48. Miller TA. Health literacy and adherence to medical treatment in chronic and acute illness: a meta-analysis. Patient Educ Couns 2016;99(7):1079–86.
49. History.com. Sully Sullenberger performs Miracle on the Hudson. Available at: https://www.history.com/this-day-in-history/sully-sullenberger-performs-miracle-on-the-hudson. Accessed June 23, 2018.

Quality Improvement Approach to Eliminate Disparities in Perinatal Morbidity and Mortality

Debra Bingham, DrPH, RN[a,b],*, David K. Jones, PhD[c],
Elizabeth A. Howell, MD, MPP[d]

KEYWORDS

- Quality improvement • Perinatal • Disparities • Maternal mortality
- Maternal morbidity • Implementation • Equity • Population health

KEY POINTS

- Women and infants of color are disproportionally affected by health care disparities.
- The Socio-Ecological Perinatal Disparities Ishikawa Diagram outlines numerous modifiable factors that can be addressed to reduce societal, community, relationship, and individual factors that contribute to perinatal disparities.
- Quality and safety principles can be used to guide national, state, and hospital-based efforts to eliminate disparities and ensure equity for all women and newborns.

INTRODUCTION

Black women are 3 to 4 times more likely to die when giving birth in the United States than white women.[1] Variation in rates of pregnancy-related death has persisted for more than 30 years and represents the greatest disparity among indicators of maternal and child health.[2,3] In a national study, case-fatality rates of black women were 2 to 3 times higher than those of white women for 5 conditions (preeclampsia, eclampsia, placenta abruption, placenta previa, and postpartum hemorrhage) even though these

Disclosure Statement: D. Bingham is the executive director of the Institute for Perinatal Quality Improvement and provides education to clinicians on the topic of increasing quality improvement and reducing perinatal disparities. She also provides consultative services.
[a] Institute for Perinatal Quality Improvement, 255 East Lombard Street, #252, Baltimore, MD 21202, USA; [b] University of Maryland School of Nursing, 344 West Lombard Street, #462A, Baltimore, MD 21201, USA; [c] Department of Health Law, Policy and Management, Boston University School of Public Health, 715 Albany Street, Boston, MA 02118, USA; [d] Department of Obstetrics, Gynecology, and Reproductive Science, Icahn School of Medicine at Mount Sinai, 1176 Fifth Avenue, Box 1170, New York, NY 10029, USA
* Corresponding author. 211 East Lombard Street, #252, Baltimore, MD 21202.
E-mail address: dbingham@perinatalQI.org

conditions were not more prevalent among black women than white women.[4] More than twice as many black women than white women (4.2% compared with 1.5%) suffered from severe morbidity at the time of birth.[5] Researchers have also shown that black women have had more inductions of labor, episiotomies, and cesarean births than white women.[6] In some cities, Hispanic women are more likely to suffer severe maternal morbidities and have higher rates of pregnancy-related death than white women.[7,8] In addition, Hispanic infants are more likely to suffer morbidities, and black infants are twice as likely to die.[9,10]

These haunting statistics clearly illustrate that disparities "are not simple differences, but rather inequities that systematically and negatively affect less advantaged groups."[11] Inequities in perinatal health care are unacceptable, and quality and safety initiatives are needed to ensure equitable care for all women and newborns. Recent data that demonstrate an increase in US maternal deaths during the past decade[12] highlight the dire need to decrease mortality and morbidity rates for all women and newborns.

A quality improvement (QI) approach has been successfully used to improve clinical outcomes, suggesting that QI can be a powerful tool to eliminating disparities. For example, universal newborn screening programs for metabolic disorders were successfully implemented in all hospitals, in all states more than 50 years ago.[13] QI initiatives have also been used to achieve outcomes that were considered highly improbable. For example, neonatal intensive care unit (NICU) leaders recently reduced the incidence of central line infections,[14] an occurrence that was previously believed to be inevitable. In fact, some NICUs have gone more than a year without central line infections. This success required careful attention to details; every step in the process was analyzed, and improvements were made as needed.

The authors propose that the following 5 quality and safety strategies should be used to guide national, state, and hospital-based efforts to eliminate disparities in perinatal outcomes and to ensure equity for all women and newborns.

STRATEGY 1: APPLY A SYSTEMS APPROACH BASED ON THE SOCIO-ECOLOGICAL MODEL

"Every system is perfectly designed to get the results it gets."[15] Our society and communities are currently perfectly designed to generate disparities in perinatal outcomes. But systems can be changed. The Socio-Ecological Model is commonly used by public health leaders to guide systems approaches to analyzing and identifying solutions to complex problems. The key insight of this framework is that a person's health is not just a function of his or her individual behaviors but also of relationships, factors present in the community, and societal context (**Fig. 1**). The Socio-Ecological Model encourages a broad, non–health care centric, systems approach to help identify the root causes of perinatal disparities.

Ishikawa cause-and-effect (fish bone) diagrams are used by quality and safety leaders to understand the key components in a system that led to a failure or contributed to a poor outcome. The Institute for Perinatal Quality Improvement used the Ishikawa diagram format and the Socio-Ecological Model to develop the Socio-Ecological Perinatal Disparities Ishikawa Diagram (**Fig. 2**). This diagram outlines numerous modifiable, system-level factors that can contribute to perinatal disparities. For example, hiring, orientation, and training practices may not be as comprehensive and may be shorter in duration for nurses among various hospitals. As a result, nurses at one hospital may be less skilled than those at another hospital, and this will affect outcomes.

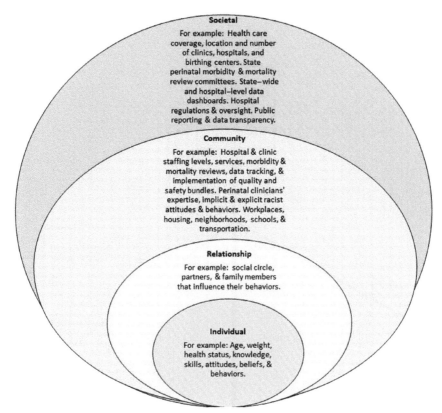

Fig. 1. Socio-Ecological Model.

Another system-level community factor is perinatal nurse staffing ratios, which vary from hospital to hospital.[16] Hospitals at which black women give birth may have lower nurse to patient ratios, thus fewer nurses are available to monitor patients, mobilize the team should a patient's condition deteriorate, provide routine care, and develop and implement QI initiatives. In a study of labor nurses, participants indicated that when they were too busy, they missed essential components of care, including complete review of the patient's history, prenatal records, and laboratory results; timely monitoring; and timely examinations.[17] These examples illustrate factors that can be modified to eliminate or greatly reduce disparities in perinatal outcomes.

STRATEGY 2: IDENTIFY ROOT CAUSES OF DISPARITIES

The first step toward reducing disparity and ensuring equity is exploring the root causes, drivers, or social determinants of perinatal disparities within our communities and facilities. A root cause analysis requires being open to learn, change, listen, and see what may not have been seen previously.

One QI approach to finding root causes is to ask "why?" multiple times. For example, if a woman is late or misses her prenatal appointment, stop and ask "why?" Do not rely solely on your assumptions. Instead, consider asking her (in a nonjudgmental way) why she was late. Consider all the barriers she may have faced to get to the appointment (eg, child care, transportation, work, school). The location

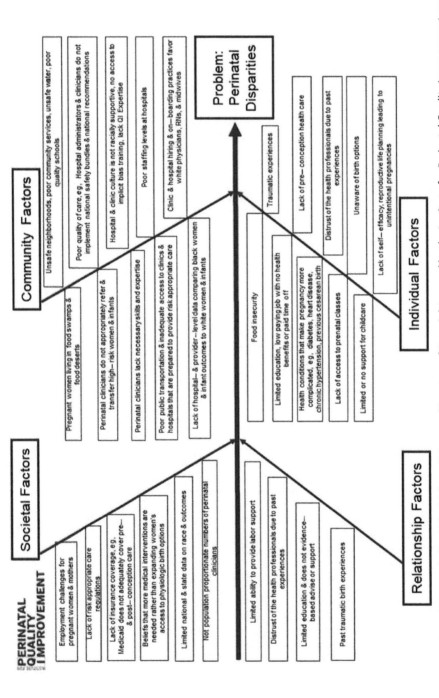

Fig. 2. Socio-Ecological Perinatal Disparities Ishikawa Diagram. (*Courtesy of* Copyright owned by the Institute for Perinatal Quality Improvement, www. perinatalQI.org, 2018, All rights reserved. Reprinted with permission.)

and hours of the clinic, public transportation schedules, and her lack of social support may affect her ability to get to the office. Similarly, it is critical to explore thoroughly the root causes of all sentinel events, near-miss events, and errors by asking "why?" A robust reporting system that encourages individuals to report, explore, and learn from poor outcomes is an effective way to identify root causes.

One major root cause of disparities is structural racism, the seen and unseen interaction among policies, practices, and institutions that perpetuate barriers preventing women and infants of color from receiving equitable and safe health care.[18] A root cause analysis can help uncover structures that contribute to disparities or inequity in the provision of care. Structural racism is perpetuated by conscious and unconscious bias and must be identified, better understood, and changed. For example, a clinician may blame black and Hispanic women for worse perinatal outcomes by assuming their behaviors reflect poor choices. However, disparities in health and health care are driven by a complex web of factors. A recent summary of epidemiologic studies about disparities in preterm birth rates concluded that place matters: not because of geography but because of systemic and structural dynamics present in social and political institutions.[19] Many more black women than white women live in "food deserts"[20] with few healthy food options or in "food swamps"[21] with limited healthy food options. In addition, higher crime rates in low-opportunity neighborhoods make it much riskier to go for a walk, play at the park, or even read a book in your own home. The cumulative effects of these negative experiences during a lifetime are not modifiable by the individual.[22]

Many clinicians routinely perpetuate structural racism. Physicians, nurses, and midwives, whose life work is dedicated to the care and healing of others, may be particularly resistant to acknowledging their roles in sustaining structural racism. Yet the facts demonstrate variation in the quality of care provided at different hospitals. For example, the risk of severe maternal morbidity at one hospital can be 6 times greater than the risk at another hospital, even after accounting for patient risk factors.[5] Not surprisingly, black and Latina women are more likely to give birth at hospitals with worse outcomes.[5] A black woman with the same risk factors as a white woman is more likely to experience severe maternal morbidity because of where she gives birth. In New York City, nearly 1000 black women could avoid severe morbidity during their birth hospitalizations each year if they gave birth at the same hospitals as white women.[5]

Numerous factors in **Fig. 2** could benefit from thorough, root cause analyses. For example, inappropriate and derogatory comments, such as "those women never take care of themselves" or "abuse the Medicaid system" are considered acceptable by some clinicians. It is important to determine the root cause of these comments and to ensure that all clinicians receive implicit bias training to prevent such comments from being made and tolerated in the future. Bias training helps clinicians become more aware of how their conscious and unconscious assumptions affect how they provide care to women of color. Bias can also manifest itself in many subtle ways, such as discounting racial and ethnic patients' symptoms or failing to adequately listen when women complain of pain. Implicit bias training was recommended by the Council on Patient Safety in Women's Healthcare as one strategy to reduce disparities because it has been shown to change attitudes and behaviors.[11]

Women of color may feel uncomfortable asking questions because of how they were previously treated by health care providers. These experiences may affect their ability to trust the current health care team. Other community factors could be explored through root cause analysis. For example, a nurse manager could explore the lack of diversity among the nurses who work on the labor and delivery unit. This root cause analysis may reveal that recruiters do not seek out graduates with diverse racial and ethnic backgrounds. Alternatively, personnel hiring and on-boarding practices may prevent a racially diverse work force, without which the team will lack different perspectives and life experiences.

STRATEGY 3: IDENTIFY AND ELIMINATE STRONG BUT WRONG ROUTINES

"Hospital quality may be a critical lever for improving outcomes and narrowing disparities."[23] All routines should be scrutinized and improved; however, a barrier to this process is that "strong but wrong routines"[24] are woven throughout clinical care. These routines are so thoroughly ingrained that it is difficult for clinicians to recognize how they contribute to deaths and injuries of women in the perinatal period. For example, for many years, estimation of blood loss at birth remained common practice despite research as early as the 1960s that demonstrated its inaccuracy.[25] In 2008, the California Maternal Quality Care Collaborative reviewed maternal deaths and pointed out that quantification of blood loss was possible and preferable. From this point, clinical practice is changing from estimation to quantification of blood loss.[26,27]

Openly discussing deaths, errors, and near-miss occurrences helps to identify structures and processes that need to be improved. Indeed, among high-reliability organizations, leaders routinely scrutinize their behavior, proactively look for potential problems, and seek to eliminate what may seem like the smallest of errors.[27] Deaths, errors, or cases of morbidity provide opportunities for learning that can lead to crucial changes. High reliability organizations establish cultures in which it is psychologically safe and desirable to discuss mistakes and proactively look for possible errors. They promote cultures that avoid blame and shame.[28]

Although individual clinicians may not have the authority to write policies for organizations, they can influence changes in practice by admitting their mistakes and identifying when a mistake was almost made irrespective of the outcome. As the Institute of Medicine emphasized, "to err is human,"[29] and no clinician is perfect. All clinicians will make mistakes at some time in their careers. The true test of clinicians' mettle is how they handle these occurrences.

Racist words and actions, just like medication errors, contribute to the preventable deaths of women and infants. Racist jokes, comments, structures, or practices may be strong but wrong routines that perpetuate a culture of disrespect and differences in how women and infants of color are cared for. These routines may be even harder to identify and change than procedure or medication errors because many are unconscious, or invisible, to individuals. Racist actions or words should be identified and addressed through reviews in the same way other health care errors are identified and reviewed.

The SPEAK UP for Black Women campaign, developed by the Institute for Perinatal Quality Improvement, encourages health care professionals (hospital administrators, clinicians, and public health leaders) to speak up against racism whenever they see racist behaviors or hear racial slurs. Individual clinicians have the power and responsibility to change the discourse (verbal, nonverbal, written) in which they participate. These types of discourse indicate the culture of an organization and how rapidly change will occur.[30] Clinicians who witness differences in care or disrespect of patients because of their race or ethnicity and do not speak up are complicit in racism. The SPEAK UP campaign encourages clinicians to receive implicit bias training and to sign the SPEAK UP pledge (**Fig. 3**).

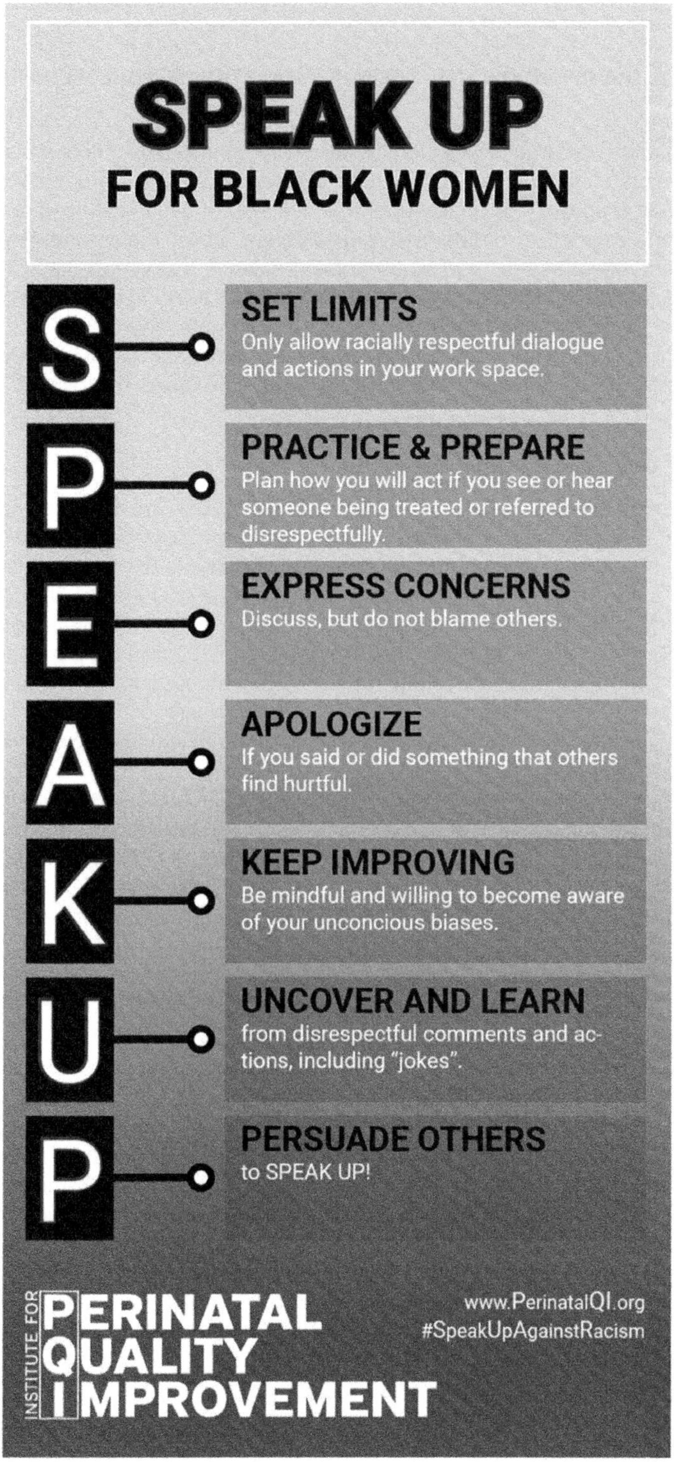

Fig. 3. The SPEAK UP campaign. (*Courtesy of* Copyright owned by the Institute for Perinatal Quality Improvement, www.perinatalQI.org, 2018, All rights reserved. Reprinted with permission.)

STRATEGY 4: USE IMPROVEMENT AND IMPLEMENTATION SCIENCE METHODS AND TOOLS

"Implementation research is the scientific study of methods to promote the systematic uptake of research findings and other evidence-based practices into routine practice, and, hence, to improve the quality and effectiveness of health services and care."[31] Improvement science is related to but different from implementation science. Improvement science is defined as an applied science that emphasizes innovation, rapid-cycle testing in the field, and spread to generate learning about what changes, in which contexts, produce improvements.[32] Implementation science and improvement science is used to guide the development, implementation, evaluation, and dissemination of QI initiatives that are designed to expand the use of evidence-based care.

Set SMART Goals and Benchmarks

QI leaders need to set goals and benchmarks. SMART goals are Specific, Measurable, Achievable, Relevant, and Time-bound. Too often the QI goals are set at 80% or 90%, rather than at 100%. Leaders and staff may also stop trying to make improvements if their goals are set too low.[33] Benchmarks with interim goals help the group track and make progress. However, once a benchmark is achieved, a new interim goal should be set until the improvements reach the ultimate goal of 100% of the population. Goals and benchmarks should be set so that they can be compared with those of other hospitals and states. Comparing outcomes in one hospital with other hospitals expands the work beyond the local context, which is often useful to identify areas in which additional improvements are needed.

QI leaders must work to ensure that vulnerable populations are included in all QI initiatives. To claim success and stop our efforts before we have made improvements for everyone leaves part of the population behind. The women and infants who are left behind may be the part of the population that needs the improvements the most. The work of quality and safety leaders is not completed until every woman and infant's outcomes are improved.

Start with Small Tests of Change Using a Quality Improvement Process Model

One of the first places to begin tackling a complex issue, such as reducing perinatal disparities, is to ensure that all women and infants have access to evidence-based interventions. These include safety protocols to standardize care, triggers, checklists, enhanced communication, and teamwork. Three QI implementation strategies used by leaders are education, discourse, and data.[34] Specific tactics can be used within each strategy. Many types of educational tactics can be used in QI initiatives. The QI leader can use academic detailing (one-on-one discussion of an academic article), classroom education, and online education. Discourse tactics can include staff meetings, bulletin board displays, and e-mails. Data tactics can include graphs, infographics with both data and images that illustrate the data, and dashboards.

Sustain Improvements

Competing priorities were identified as a significant threat to sustaining the gains of a QI initiative.[35] Whenever the QI leaders begin to introduce new QI initiatives, they also need to perform periodic surveillance because it is important to know whether the previous successes are being sustained. Effective continual surveillance provides alerts. Ongoing surveillance is particularly important when working to reduce long-standing perinatal disparities.

STRATEGY 5: USE DATA TO GUIDE THE PLAN AND TRACK PROGRESS

Data form the foundation of system thinking, root cause analyses, and QI methods. QI leaders need to be thoroughly informed about how data are collected and presented to ensure that no racial group or ethnicity is risk adjusted out of their hospital's QI data. Data variation is how QI leaders identify opportunities for improvement.

Donabedian's[36] structure, process, and outcomes QI data measurement categories are a practical way to use and categorize data to guide QI efforts. These data categories are useful when developing the QI metrics to assess, plan, and track QI progress. Balancing measures, especially when working to make improvements in maternal outcomes, also may be needed. It is important to have a balance between maternal and neonatal measures to ensure that a QI effort designed to reduce cesarean births, for example, does not lead to negative, unintended consequences for the infants.

Structural changes, such as improving an electronic health record, developing a new policy and procedure, or providing education for the clinical staff, make it easier for clinicians to do the right thing. Structural changes are especially necessary when working to eliminate perinatal disparities. For example, ensuring that more women and men of color are admitted to medical and nursing schools and are hired to work in the outpatient and inpatient settings is a needed change. Only by achieving a diverse workforce will we be able to serve the needs of our ever-increasing diversity of patients. Further, unconscious bias training needs to be implemented in medical schools, nursing schools, and hospitals to help recognize our own biases and serve our patients better. Structural changes that will reduce disparities could include more convenient clinic hours, making it more accessible for the most vulnerable populations or implementing implicit bias training. Structural changes may be the changes that take the longest to make, but structural changes are worth the effort because they are the hardest to circumvent.

Process measures, such as quantification of blood loss, performing risk assessments, and accurately taking a blood pressure, are focused on changing clinicians' behaviors. Examples of a disparity-related process measure is to implement more respectful dialogue among the clinicians, change hiring practices, and change onboarding practices. Outlining examples of what is and is not respectful speech and actions and performing role playing are tactics that can be used to successfully implement these process improvements.

Rates of severe maternal morbidity and mortality are an example of an outcome measure. Data need to be analyzed and presented in such a way that any differences in outcomes by race and ethnicity are easy to identify. QI data need to be designed so that outcomes of different racial and ethnic groups can be easily compared within a hospital, across hospitals, communities, regions, and nationally. Hospital-level severe maternal morbidity data showed a wide variation in black women compared with white women.[5] These data provide the opportunity for further explorations. For example, the hospitals with the highest rates of severe maternal mortality should perform a formal root cause analysis to determine why their rates are higher than other hospitals. In addition, there also can be disparities within the same hospital.[5] Knowing the differences in severe maternal morbidity for black women compared with white women, especially if the black women gave birth at the same hospital as the white women, will help support the root cause analysis that will guide the development and implementation of a targeted QI initiative. Recording race and ethnicity birth data as accurately as possible is a recommendation from the Council on Patient Safety and is critical to the success of QI efforts designed to eliminate preventable disparities.[11]

SUMMARY

A disproportionate number of women and infants of color are suffering preventable harm in the United States resulting in the premature loss of life. These losses create a cascade of negative effects across multiple generations. Each maternal death can result in grandmothers, grandfathers, aunts, uncles, friends, and communities stepping in to raise a motherless child. Each loss of a child results in excruciating and life-long pain for mothers, fathers, and families. These premature losses put families of color at a disadvantage over the life-course.

More than half of maternal deaths are preventable.[37–39] We must act now to increase our QI capacity if we are to reduce the 17-year lag time between knowing and doing.[40] Applying QI principles to the complex, multifaceted goal of ensuring perinatal equity for all women is an important start to mapping out and implementing a course of action. When trying to resolve complex issues and make important changes, we can be energized and encouraged by what Margaret Meade said: "never doubt that a small group of thoughtful, committed citizens can change the world; indeed, it's the only thing that ever has."[41]

REFERENCES

1. Creanga AA, Syverson C, Seed K, et al. Pregnancy-related mortality in the United States, 2011-2013. Obstet Gynecol 2017;130(2):366–73.
2. Centers for Disease Control and Prevention. Differences in maternal mortality among black and white women - United States, 1990. MMWR Morb Mortal Wkly Rep 1995;44(1):6–7, 13–14. Available at: https://www.cdc.gov/mmwr/preview/mmwrhtml/00035538.htm. Accessed October 12, 2018.
3. Berg CJ, Chang J, Callaghan WM, et al. Pregnancy-related mortality in the United States, 1991-1997. Obstet Gynecol 2003;101(2):289–96. Available at: https://journals.lww.com/greenjournal/Fulltext/2003/02000/Pregnancy_Related_Mortality_in_the_United_States,.15.aspx. Accessed October 12, 2018.
4. Tucker MJ, Berg CJ, Callaghan WM, et al. The black-white disparity in pregnancy-related mortality from 5 conditions: differences in prevalence and case-fatality rates. Am J Public Health 2007;97(2):247–51.
5. Howell EA, Egorova NN, Balbierz A, et al. Site of delivery contribution to black-white severe maternal morbidity disparity. Am J Obstet Gynecol 2016;215(2):143–52.
6. Grobman WA, Bailit JL, Rice MM, et al. Racial and ethnic disparities in maternal morbidity and obstetric care. Obstet Gynecol 2015;125(6):1460–7.
7. Howell EA, Egorova NN, Janevic T, et al. Severe maternal morbidity among Hispanic women in New York City: investigation of health disparities. Obstet Gynecol 2017;129(2):285–94.
8. New York City Department of Health and Mental Hygiene. Severe maternal morbidity in New York City, 2008–2012 2016. Avaialable at: https://www1.nyc.gov/assets/doh/downloads/pdf/data/maternal-morbidity-report-08-12.pdf. Accessed September 28, 2018.
9. Howell EA, Janevic T, Hebert PL, et al. Differences in morbidity and mortality rates in black, white, and Hispanic very preterm infants among New York City hospitals. JAMA Pediatr 2018;172(3):269–77.
10. Matthews TJ, MacDorman MF, Thoma ME. Infant mortality statistics from the 2013 period linked birth/infant death data set. Natl Vital Stat Rep 2015;64(9):1–30. Avaialable at: https://www.cdc.gov/nchs/data/nvsr/nvsr64/nvsr64_09.pdf. Accessed October 12, 2018.

11. Howell EA, Brown H, Brumley J, et al. Reduction of peripartum racial and ethnic disparities: a conceptual framework and maternal safety consensus bundle. J Obstet Gynecol Neonatal Nurs 2018;47:275–86.

12. GBD 2015 Maternal Mortality Collaborators. Global, regional, and national levels of maternal mortality, 1990-2015: a systematic analysis for the Global Burden of Disease Study 2015. Lancet 2016;388(10053):1775–812.

13. Brosco J, Grosse S, Ross L. Universal state newborn screening programs can reduce health disparities. JAMA Pediatr 2015;169(1):7–8.

14. Mobley RE, Bizzarro MJ. Central line-associated bloodstream infections in the NICU: successes and controversies in the quest for zero. Semin Perinatol 2017;41(3):166–74.

15. IHI Multimedia Team. Like magic? ("Every system is perfectly designed..."). 2015. Available at: https://www.ihi.org/communities/blogs/origin-of-every-system-is-perfectly-designed-quote. Accessed September 9, 2018.

16. Scheich B, Bingham D. Key Findings from the AWHONN perinatal staffing data collaborative. J Obstet Gynecol Neonatal Nurs 2015;44(2):317–28.

17. Simpson KR, Lyndon A. Consequences of delayed, unfinished, or missed nursing care during labor and birth. J Perinat Neonatal Nurs 2017;31(1):32–40.

18. Bailey ZD, Krieger N, Agénor M, et al. Structural racism and health inequities in the USA: evidence and interventions. Lancet 2017;389(10077). https://doi.org/10.1016/S0140-6736(17)30569-X.

19. Lu MC. Place matters to birth outcomes: a life-course perspective. Paediatr Perinat Epidemiol 2018. https://doi.org/10.1111/ppe.12498.

20. Cummins S, Macintyre S. "Food deserts" — evidence and assumption in health policy making. BMJ 2002;325(7361):436–8. Avaialable at: https://www.ncbi.nlm.nih.gov/pubmed/12193363.

21. Rose D, Bodor JN, Swalm CM, et al. Deserts in New Orleans? Illustrations of urban food access and implications for policy. Avaialable at: https://pdfs.semanticscholar.org/abc8/b418aa0783c8f3b0a0c4fca8f137ad806e0a.pdf. Accessed October 9, 2018.

22. Lu MC, Halfon N. Racial and ethnic disparities in birth outcomes: a life-course perspective. Matern Child Health J 2003;7(1):13–30.

23. Howell EA, Zeitlin J. Improving hospital quality to reduce disparities in severe maternal morbidity and mortality. Semin Perinatol 2017;41(5):266–72.

24. Reason J. Human error. Manchester (England): Cambridge University Press; 1990. p. 21.

25. Main EK, Goffman D, Scavone BM, et al. National partnership for maternal safety: consensus bundle on obstetric hemorrhage. J Obstet Gynecol Neonatal Nurs 2015;44(4):462–70.

26. Bingham D, Lyndon A, Lagrew D, et al. A state-wide obstetric hemorrhage quality improvement initiative. MCN Am J Matern Child Nurs 2011;36(5):297–304.

27. Bingham D. Applying the generic errors modeling system to obstetric hemorrhage quality improvement efforts. J Obstet Gynecol Neonatal Nurs 2012;41(4):540–50.

28. Weick KE, Sutcliffe KM. Managing the unexpected: assuring high performance in an age of complexity. San Francsico (CA): Jossey-Bass; 2001.

29. Institute of Medicine. To err is human: building a safer health system. 1999. Avaialble at: http://www.nationalacademies.org/hmd/~/media/Files/Report%20Files/1999/To-Err-is-Human/To%20Err%20is%20Human%201999%20%20report%20brief.pdf. Accessed October 8, 2018.

30. Ford JD, Ford LW. Conversations and the authoring of change. In: Holman D, Thorpe R, editors. Management and language: the manager as a practical author. London: SAGE Publications; 2003. p. 141–57.
31. Eccles MP, Mittman BS. Welcome to implementation science. Implement Sci 2006;1(1):1–3.
32. Institute for Healthcare Improvement. Science of improvement. Available at: http://www.ihi.org/about/Pages/ScienceofImprovement.aspx. Accessed October 9, 2018.
33. Bingham D. Setting perinatal quality and safety goals: should we strive for best outcomes. Midwifery 2010;26(5):483–4.
34. Bingham D, Main EK. Effective implementation strategies and tactics for leading change on maternity units. J Perinat Neonatal Nurs 2010;24(1):32–42.
35. Seacrist M, Bingham D, Scheich B, et al. Barriers and facilitators to implementation of a multistate collaborative to reduce maternal mortality from postpartum hemorrhage. J Obstet Gynecol Neonatal Nurs 2018;47(5):688–97.
36. Donabedian A. Evaluating the quality of medical care. Milbank Q 2005;83(4): 691–729.
37. Berg CJ, Harper MA, Atkinson SM, et al. Preventability of pregnancy-related deaths: results of a state-wide review. Obstet Gynecol 2005;106(6):1228–34.
38. Della Torre M, Kilpatrick SJ, Hibbard JU, et al. Assessing preventability for obstetric hemorrhage. Am J Perinatol 2011;28(10):753–60.
39. Wong CA, Scott S, Jones RL, et al. The State of Illinois obstetric hemorrhage project: pre-project and post-training examination scores. J Matern Fetal Neonatal Med 2016;29(5):845–9.
40. Institute of Medicine. Crossing the quality chasm: a new health system for the 21st century. Avaialble at: https://www.nap.edu/catalog/10027/crossing-the-quality-chasm-a-new-health-system-for-the. Accessed October 12, 2018.
41. Lutkehaus NC. Margaret Mead: the making of an American icon. Princeton (NJ): Princeton University Press; 2008.

Focus on Culture

Patient Safety and the Just Culture

David Marx, BSE, JD*

KEYWORDS

- Just Culture • Human error • At-risk behavior • Patient safety

KEY POINTS

- By creating the psychological safety for physicians to report errors, Just Culture is a cornerstone of patient safety.
- Just Culture uses common language to consistently and fairly evaluate physician behavior.
- Just Culture shifts the focus from errors and outcomes to system design and behavioral choices.
- Just Culture creates a culture of accountability; it is not punitive, nor blame free.

INTRODUCTION

In 2000, Dr Lucian Leape, considered by many to be the father of the modern patient safety movement, testified before Congress:

> The single greatest impediment to patient safety is that we punish people for making mistakes.[1]

Dr Leape went on to say that in his physician culture, practitioners would report only what they could not hide. Lucian's testimony reflected a sentiment thought within many high-consequence industries. Aviation long worked under the code of "what happened in the cockpit stays in the cockpit." Pilots did not feel comfortable coming forward with their errors or observations of unsafe systems. In aviation, creating learning cultures had taken a backseat to the sport of blame. Something goes wrong, point the finger of blame, take disciplinary and enforcement action, convince ourselves that the culprit has been caught, and the problem is solved.

Disclosure Statement: D. Marx is the owner and CEO of Outcome Engenuity, which produces Just Culture materials used by high-risk industries around the world.
Outcome Engenuity
* 5048 Tennyson Parkway, Suite 250, Plano, TX 75024.
E-mail address: dmarx@outcome-eng.com

Obstet Gynecol Clin N Am 46 (2019) 239–245
https://doi.org/10.1016/j.ogc.2019.01.003
obgyn.theclinics.com

Aviation safety specialists around the world could see the problem with this blame-the-last-person-who-touched-it approach. As in health care, critical safety information was concealed; potentially deadly errors were destined to repeat themselves.

By the 1970s, aviation safety specialists began creating blame-free, nonpunitive reporting programs. On behalf of the Federal Aviation Administration (FAA), NASA's Aviation Safety Reporting System offered an enforcement-related incentive to pilots who voluntarily reported safety-critical information.[2] In the 1990s, the FAA worked further to foster internal airline reporting programs under its Aviation Safety Action Programs, where individual pilots could report near misses to event review teams comprising FAA, airline, and pilot union personnel.[3]

Learning from aviation, health care followed suit with Congress passing the Patient Safety Act of 2008. Its Patient Safety Organization provisions created a safe space for health care providers to report what they might otherwise hide. Internally, hospital administrators also worked hard to convince staff to report safety critical information. "Nonpunitive, blame-free" reporting was the talk of the town.

Just Culture was a concept with different ideological roots. Open reporting was a similar goal; yet, creating rules requiring perfection and then offering immunity for those who fell short did not seem to be the ideal path. Would we need safe havens for reporting if we could simply treat people justly? Did it really make sense to make our inescapable fallibility a crime in the first place? In addition, did "blame-free" really do anything to change routine risky behavior? If a surgeon did not want to participate in a presurgical timeout, was a nonpunitive reporting program likely to help?

Just Culture became the alternative, focused not exclusively on nonpunitive reporting, but instead on a proper human-centered system of accountability. Could we create a system of workplace justice that fostered open reporting, while simultaneously holding people appropriately accountable for their actions? Could we move past safe havens for reporting, to create a set of human resource standards that would allow an employee to report right to their supervisor or chief? That was the challenge for the Just Culture.

FINDING THE RIGHT LANGUAGE
Malpractice, Medical Error, Disruptive Behavior, Negligence, Unprofessional Conduct

There are a variety of terms used to describe undesired conduct and the outcomes that result. All of the terms have some level of negative connotation, expressing a level of falling short, if not outright blame and shame. We might hear that British Petroleum was negligent in the Gulf of Mexico's Deepwater Horizon disaster. It tells us little, technically, but it oozes condemnation.

Through Just Culture, organizations have attempted to address this general lack of precision, and its attendant confusion. It starts with getting a handle on the idea of "intention." The phrase, "but she did not intend to harm the patient," might be correct, but it does not fully describe what was going on. Our brains create 2 intentions for each of our behaviors:– the intention toward the act itself, and the intention toward the outcome. A physician may choose to skip a procedurally required step, but not the risk of harm they take. Intention must be understood beyond the question of whether the provider "intended" harm. Borrowing from the model penal code,[4] 4 slightly more sophisticated levels of intention are identified (**Fig. 1**).

Purpose
Purpose is the choice to act, with the express goal of causing harm.

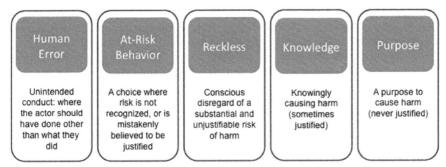

Human Error	At-Risk Behavior	Reckless	Knowledge	Purpose
Unintended conduct: where the actor should have done other than what they did	A choice where risk is not recognized, or is mistakenly believed to be justified	Conscious disregard of a substantial and unjustifiable risk of harm	Knowingly causing harm (sometimes justified)	A purpose to cause harm (never justified)

Fig. 1. The 5 behaviors. (Copyright Outcome Engenuity 2017.)

Knowledge

Knowledge is the choice to act, knowing that harm is practically certain to occur. It should be noted that sometimes harm is the right answer, if it is the lesser of 2 evils. This, however, is the exception. Knowingly causing harm is generally a very culpable act.

Reckless

Technically, recklessness is the conscious disregard of a substantial and unjustifiable risk. It is not an intention to cause harm, but merely the willingness to accept an unjustifiable risk. It is most easily viewed as "gambling" toward the possible outcome. It is to put personal interest ahead of an unjustifiable risk of harm to others. The reckless person does not intend the outcome; they just choose the gamble.

Negligence

Negligence relates to the risk that a person should have been aware of, but was not. It is the same substantial and unjustifiable risk from the definition of reckless, but rather than conscious disregard, there is no conscious choice to take the unjustifiable risk. However, those who stand in judgment determine that, under the circumstances, the person should have been aware of the risk.

These are the 4 levels of intention that legal scholars can provide to us: Purpose, knowledge, reckless, and negligence. There is, however, an operational problem with the latter term, "negligence." The problem with negligence is that its street definition is very different from its legal definition. Legally, it targets the notion that an actor should have been aware but was unaware of a substantial and unjustifiable risk. This negligence is where most medical malpractice, and most human error, resides. No evil intention, no unjustifiable risk taking. In contrast, the street definition of negligence usually involves some level of indifference, or evil intention.

In the Just Culture model, negligence is split into 2 distinct behaviors. The first is at-risk behavior, the choice to engage the behavior, but being unaware of the unjustifiable risk. The second is human error, where the behavior itself is not chosen. Human error involves all of those actions we did not choose to do, like mistakenly writing an incorrect order, or a misread of a fetal heart tracing. At-risk behaviors are the routine choices that add risk, but with the risk not being seen by the provider. Examples might include a choice not to ask 2-patient identifiers, or a choice to rapidly proceed through a history and physical examination of a familiar patient.

Purpose; Knowledge; Reckless; at-risk behavior; human error: each term has precision, and each level of culpability has its own causes and its own solutions. For most of us, however, justice is both intellectual and emotional. Not everyone is an obstetrician, and not everyone is an astronaut; however, we are all judges. We all watch how the organization reacts to each of these. Was an obstetrician sanctioned for an inescapable human error? Is the disruptive behavior of the gynecologist being ignored by the organization? How a society, how an organization, and how a peer-review panel react to each of these levels of intention will shape the views of workplace justice.

THE SEVERITY BIAS

On good days, we evaluate each other's conduct based on intent. On bad days, it is often about outcome. This effect is particularly true for the miracle of childbirth. After 9 months of care for their unborn child, mothers and fathers expect a pretty good outcome on the day of delivery. Experience a bad outcome, and everyone is looking for the person to blame.

There is a flip side to this coin. It is called "no harm, no foul." Perhaps it is our attachment to liberty, or our natural conflict avoidance, but whatever the reason, we culturally give one another grace when our risky choices do not lead to harm. As a physician, if you cut a corner to get a good outcome, you are the hero. Cut that same corner, create a bad outcome, and you will likely be vilified.

Central to the concept of Just Culture is the shift away from outcome, to a focus on behavioral choices. Putting it bluntly, luck is the only difference between the drunk driver who kills and the one who does not. Skipping a presurgical timeout and then justifying it based on the fact there was no bad outcome ignores the probabilistic link between choices and outcomes. Whether a patient lives or dies may mark the difference between success and tragedy. Justice, in contrast, should be blind to the actual outcome. If a physician's conduct is being assessed in peer review, the focus should rightly be placed on the quality of the provider's choices rather than the harm that those choices produced.

THROWING OUT THE BABY WITH THE BATHWATER

"No one comes to work intending to cause harm," CEOs have said. Patient Safety Officers nod their heads in agreement. Human Resource Officers know the truth.

For CEOs, saying this aspiration is part of the marketing pitch around the need to have employees report unsafe conditions and the errors that they cause. Fixing bad systems is the message. For Patient Safety officers, their entire game is played at the lower end of the culpability spectrum. Human error, at-risk behavior, and the occasionally reckless are the scope of their practice. People generally do come to work to do the right thing. When things do not go as planned, it is generally because of a poorly designed system, say the Patient Safety officers.

To create more open reporting, we need not say that all undesired outcomes are unintended. CEOs need not tell their teams that all unintended outcomes are caused by bad system design. To create a learning culture, we need not throw personal accountability out the window, nor should we. For clinical chiefs and the Human Resource Officer, there remains a sea of behavior at the other end of the culpability spectrum. The Joint Commission's Sentinel Event Alert on Disruptive Behavior, and more recently, the #MeToo movement highlight that it is not only human errors that concern us.[5] Occasionally, providers engage in highly culpable behavior. They will look into a patient's clinical record when they are not the care providers; they will use inappropriate or offensive language toward coworkers, and they will on occasion steal drugs for their own drug habit. It is not conduct exclusive to providers; rather, it is conduct that makes us all human. In addition, physician leaders, like all leaders, will occasionally engage in behavior that we have societally condemned, from not hiring or not promoting because of gender, race, or religion, to sexual harassment and assault. Self-centered creatures that we are, we will sometimes put our own interests ahead of others, risking or knowingly causing harm.

Both ends of the culpability spectrum must be addressed in a Just Culture. Although patient safety focuses on the human error and at-risk behaviors, many people's view of workplace justice stems from perceived unjust responses to discrimination or unprofessional behavior. For Just Culture to work, it must address the full spectrum of human behavior.

THE JUST CULTURE MODEL

The 5 following behaviors may result in harm:

- Human error
- At-risk behavior
- Reckless behavior
- Knowledge toward virtually certain harm
- Deliberately seeking to cause harm

All behaviors are qualitatively different, and all behaviors are technically and legally different. The Just Culture views these 5 behaviors as operationally different behaviors. In simple form, a more "just" culture might promote the following:

- Accept the error
- Coach the at-risk behavior
- Sanction the reckless, knowledge, and purpose (**Fig. 2**)

Accept the Error

Human error is unintended. We do not choose human error; it happens to us, shaped by the systems in which we work, and choices we make it those systems. In this context, it is best to think of human error as an outcome rather than a conduct. To accept the error is to refrain from any sanction, and to turn our attention to the systems and choices that might have led to the error.

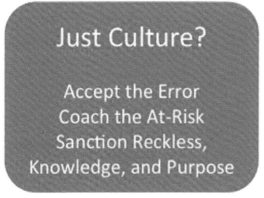

Fig. 2. The just culture model. (Copyright Outcome Engenuity 2017.)

Coach the At-Risk Behavior

At-risk behavior is defined as a risky choice, but where the individual does not see the risk, or incorrectly thinks the risk is justified. Coaching, in this context, is a discussion about the risks associated with the behavior. It need not only be manager/subordinate. Coaching can be a peer-to-peer conversation about the pros and cons of a particular behavioral choice.

Sanction the Reckless, Knowledge, and Purpose

We leave the threat of sanction to more culpable behaviors. Threat is a provocative word in this circumstance, but used precisely to address the unique role of sanction. Sanction is a form of artificial danger. If evidence shows that we humans do not see the harm in a particular course of conduct, we might societally attach artificial danger to the conduct. Privacy laws in health care did just that by creating criminal penalties for a decision to invade a patient's private health information. Likewise, if a provider does not recognize her language as offensive, she may see the organizational threat of sanction to be enough to choose a less offensive communication style.

So how do these 5 behaviors work in a Just Culture? As an example, consider the following scenario: An obstetrician loudly and publicly berates a nurse in the hallway because the nurse had misunderstood a previous instruction. Now distraught, the nurse, with medication in hand, proceeds into the room right in front of him and gives the medication to the wrong patient. Neither the nurse nor the obstetrician intended any harm to the patient. Under the Just Culture, the events would be analyzed as follows: The nurse gave the patient a drug that did not belong to the patient (the undesired outcome). The nurse walked into the wrong room (a human error). The nurse, befuddled by the physician's berating, unintentionally skips the 2-patient identifier check (human error). The obstetrician berates the nurse (the at-risk or reckless choice toward the patient). Determination of whether the obstetrician's conduct was at risk or reckless toward the patient depends on how the collective culture sees the risk of patient harm from disruptive behavior. If it is not tolerated within the culture because the culture sees it as potentially harmful to patients, it would likely be seen as reckless. There is, of course, in this scenario, a second harm, that being the direct harm to the nurse. In this case, the obstetrician's behavior might easily be seen as knowingly harmful to the nurse, because the berating conduct was not aligned with the value of respect held within the organization (**Fig. 3**).

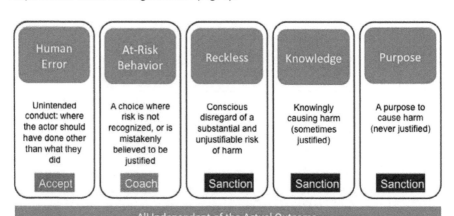

Fig. 3. Just response to the 5 behaviors. (Copyright Outcome Engenuity 2017.)

Address the Repetitive

Beyond the single event, a Just Culture should address repetitive behavior. In particular, both human errors and at-risk behaviors can be repetitive in a manner that might warrant a different response than to accept or coach. At some point, we may find a provider that looks like an outlier. It could be the provider that we see as a mistake waiting to happen, or the provider who is resistant to coaching around a particular behavioral choice. If a high rate of error cannot be remedied, the error-prone provider might need to be removed from a place of potential harm. Likewise, if a provider is not amenable to coaching, there may be a need to progress to some form of disciplinary action.

THE BENEFITS OF A JUST CULTURE

By adopting a Just Culture, an organization can shift its focus from judging errors and outcomes to focusing on their origins. They can move beyond "how bad was the outcome, and who did it?" to a much more productive discussion about system design and behavioral choices. By being just, we create a much more open learning culture, allowing us to fix bad systems around good providers. As an example, Magruder Hospital in Port Clinton, Ohio, spent 6 years on its journey to a more "just" culture. From 2012 to 2018, their Agency for Healthcare Research and Quality (AHRQ) Patient Safety Survey percent-positive composite score for nonpunitive response to errors moved from 36% to 77%.[6,7] This resulting score is 30% points above the 2018 national hospital average of 47%. In addition, Magruder reports improvement across all AHRQ patient safety survey measures.

For individual providers, we create a psychologically safer environment in which to practice medicine. The Just Culture provides clinical chiefs and peer reviewers a more rational basis for evaluating the conduct of providers. We take the expectation of perfection off the table and replace it with the goal of safe choices, something much more achievable for individual providers. In doing so, we create more accountability rather than less.

By being more just, we create better outcomes for the patients and families we serve.

REFERENCES

1. S. HRG, 106-847, Medical Mistakes, Joint Hearing before the Subcommittee on Labor Health and Human Services, 2001.
2. Federal Aviation Administration Advisory Circular AC 00-666E - Aviation Safety Reporting Program, December 16, 2011.
3. Federal Aviation Administration Advisory Circular AC 120-66B - Aviation Safety Action Program (ASAP), November 15, 2002.
4. American Law Institute. Model Penal Code, 2.02 general requirements of culpability. Washington, DC: American Law Institute; 1962.
5. Joint Commission. Sentinel event alert issue 40: behaviors that undermine a culture of safety 2008. Available at: https://www.jointcommission.org/sentinel_event_alert_issue_40_behaviors_that_undermine_a_culture_of_safety/. Accessed June 1, 2018.
6. Marsico N, Oman L, Marx D. Interview: a just culture conversation with the leadership of Magruder Hospital 2018. Available at: https://youtu.be/Lb7XtlZRLtk. Accessed June 1, 2018.
7. Agency for Healthcare Research and Quality. Patient safety survey 2004. Available at: https://www.ahrq.gov/sops/quality-patient-safety/patientsafetyculture/hospital/index.html. Accessed June 1, 2018.

Transparency and Disclosure

Jonathan L. Gleason, MD[a,b,*], Eric Swisher, MD[b,1],
Patrice M. Weiss, MD[a,b]

KEYWORDS

• Transparency • Disclosure • Early resolution • Patient safety • Medical error

KEY POINTS

- Medical errors and adverse events are common.
- Medical errors and adverse events should be disclosed to patients.
- There are techniques that ensure a disclosure is performed well.
- Disclosure of medical errors facilitates improvement in patient safety.

CASE STUDY

During a busy night on labor and delivery at a tertiary care hospital, a patient with pre-eclampsia was being induced at term. Her blood pressures were managed and she was administered magnesium sulfate for seizure prophylaxis. As she reached the second stage of labor, the patient experienced a seizure. During treatment of her seizure, fetal bradycardia occurred. The fetal heart rate did not recover after the mother was stabilized. A "STAT" cesarean section was performed. The baby survived and was left with severe neurologic impairment. The mother also suffered a stroke and was left with mild persistent neurologic impairment. During the event, it was discovered that the magnesium sulfate level was significantly subtherapeutic at the time of delivery. It was suspected that the infusion had not been running, although the reasons were unclear. Many difficult questions arise regarding if, when, and how to share this information with the patient.

There have been medical errors and unexpected outcomes for as long as there has been medical care. The practice of medicine is inherently dangerous and complex. For much of the twentieth century in the United States, hospitals and medical malpractice defense attorneys generally promoted a strategy referred to as "deny and defend."[1] This strategy to reduce and avoid exposure encouraged providers and staff to avoid disclosing medical errors. There are numerous reasons why this strategy was

Disclosure Statement: The authors have no financial disclosures.
[a] Carilion Clinic, 1906 Belleview Avenue, SE, Roanoke, VA 24014, USA; [b] Virginia Tech Carilion School of Medicine, 902 South Jefferson Street, Roanoke, VA 24016, USA
[1] Present address: 21 Highland Avenue, Southeast Suite 200, Roanoke, VA 24013.
* Corresponding author. Carilion Clinic, 1906 Belleview Avenue, SE, Roanoke, VA 24014.
E-mail address: jlgleason@carilionclinic.org

recommended. Defense attorneys know that a very small proportion of potentially compensable events are ever compensated. They postulate that this is true because patients were never clearly made aware of the error.[2] Disclosure of errors was thought to increase exposure to medical malpractice claims. Defense attorneys also know that more than half of all malpractice claims that are brought against doctors and hospitals in the United States are ultimately abandoned by plaintiffs. Many claims are abandoned during the discovery phase when defense counsel works deliberately to avoid disclosing damaging facts. Thus the idea of disclosing "bad facts" is antithetical to their strategy in defending a medical malpractice claim. Beginning in 2007, there has been a rapid move away from "deny and defend" toward a strategy of transparency, apology, and disclosure of medical errors.

There are many reasons why this change has occurred. We live in a very different world in the twenty-first century, where several factors have come together to topple "deny and defend" as the singular strategy for managing adverse outcomes in health care.

WIDESPREAD ACKNOWLEDGMENT OF PERVASIVE ERRORS AND HARM IN HEALTH CARE

To Err is Human: *Building a Safer Health System*, published in November 1999 by the Institute of Medicine, estimated that 98,000 people die every year from medical errors.[3] This report significantly contributed to the push for large-scale change in health care, including electronic health records, pay-for-performance, and transparency regarding hospital outcomes. Local and national media have rightly focused much attention on these disturbing reports, and routinely report on medical errors. Groups such as Leap-Frog also promote the measurement of safety and harm at hospitals. Sadly, the National Patient Safety Foundation Report, *Not Enough Change Since To Err is Human*, reported that very little progress had been made in reducing errors and harm in health care in 2015.[4] Even more recently, researchers at Johns Hopkins Medicine reported that medical errors are the third leading cause of death in the United States.[5] Consequently, patients have a greater awareness of the potential for harm, are more vigilant, and are less likely to assume that their care was safe and appropriate.

REGULATORY AGENCIES REQUIRING DISCLOSURE OF ADVERSE EVENTS OR OUTCOMES

Following *To Err is Human*, in 2001 the Joint Commission (TJC) sought to make disclosure of unanticipated outcomes a requirement for hospitals.[6] Since that time, 10 states have mandated disclosure of unanticipated outcomes to patients.

TECHNOLOGY HAS CREATED A GREATER EXPECTATION OF TRANSPARENCY

The Internet combined with the broad availability of consumer feedback has created the expectation of total transparency. The public demands information about every aspect of their life in order to make informed decisions such as purchasing vacuum cleaners, hiring plumbers, and catching a ride. The public increasingly demands total access to information at all times and is less tolerant of opacity around cost and safety in health care.

RAPID INCREASE IN HEALTH CARE COST

The United States spent $3.7 trillion on health care in 2018.[7] The average price of an outpatient office visit increased 69% from 2003 to 2016 in large employer health plans, far outpacing the 28% increase in overall inflation over the same time period. The average price of laparoscopic appendectomy procedures increased 136% over this period, from $8570 to $20,192.[8]

The general awareness of pervasive preventable harm and escalating costs, paired with a general expectation of transparency, has contributed to the move toward greater transparency in health care.

FOUNDATIONS OF TRANSPARENCY AND DISCLOSURE IN MEDICINE
Why?

Most would agree that there is a moral imperative to be truthful about medical errors and adverse outcomes that result in serious harm. The Code of Medical Ethics of the American Medical Association states that "physicians should at all times deal honestly and openly with patients."[9] Honesty and transparency are simply fundamental to moral human interactions, including the practice of medicine. Some physicians have postulated that patients may not want to be made aware of every mistake, but this notion is contradictory to evidence that patients would like to have full knowledge of errors that occur during their care, regardless of the severity of the harm.[10] Furthermore, providers may suffer moral distress when withholding errors from patients. Labor and delivery staff may suffer ongoing guilt and shame if they are unable to explain to their unfortunate patient what occurred with the magnesium sulfate infusion in the aforementioned case.

The more significant benefit of disclosure is that it facilitates a more robust response to errors and increases the speed at which process changes can occur to prevent harm in other patients.[11–15] There is evidence that one of the primary motivations of patients to file medical malpractice lawsuits is to learn the truth. They are angry, feeling that information was withheld.[10] Several health systems have committed to total transparency and have implemented programs to compensate patients who suffer harm from medical errors. These early-resolution programs report overall reductions in medical malpractice claims expenditure and a more expedient resolution with patients.[16] Transparency and disclosure is the first step in facilitating early resolution of medical errors in a way that supports both the health system and the patients.

Creating a comprehensive program for identifying medical errors or adverse outcomes is an essential first step in transparency. Event reporting should then be used to facilitate disclosure of errors and adverse outcomes. To do this consistently, practices and health systems must have a well-trained provider group who value disclosure as well as a comprehensive implementation program. The governing board and medical leadership must develop policies that clearly articulate and support a transparency and safety culture.

What?

There is consensus among regulatory agencies such as TJC that medical errors resulting in serious harm must be disclosed. Controversy remains regarding disclosure of medical errors that do not result in serious harm. It is estimated that more than 1 million medical errors occur annually in the United States, many of which are not reported.[10] It is difficult to measure disclosures of errors that did not result in serious harm because such events may not be reported. Adverse outcomes for some errors, such as diagnostic errors, may not be immediately apparent. It is therefore less confusing and more consistent with the wishes of our patients to disclose all known errors irrespective of clinical outcomes or harm.

Who?

TJC specifically states that the attending physician, or their designee, should disclose unanticipated outcomes of care, treatment, and services related to sentinel events.[17] This recommendation is consistent with maintaining the physician-patient relationship during an unexpected outcome. However, the provider may not be able to discuss the event because of distress or grief. If the provider is not able to disclose an error in a timely manner, a partner who is involved with the management of the patient is a reasonable designee. For events that result in serious harm, for example in the aforementioned case study, it is recommended that providers consult with Clinical Risk Management at their institution, who may help the provider to appropriately disclose the event. Each state has specific laws and precedent that may inform best practices for disclosure. It may be helpful to include other members of the health team if appropriate (eg, nursing). It is recommended that the group disclosing the error should be outnumbered by the patient and their family members during the discussion. The patient and her family should not feel overwhelmed. Disclosure should be regarded as an act of honest humility rather than a show of force. It is not recommended to include high-level hospital administration in the initial disclosure.

Disclosure of less serious events by all members of the health care team occurs routinely during medical care. Failure to send a refill prescription in a timely manner, for example, may be disclosed by nursing staff at the physician's office. This type of behavior should be encouraged, modeled, and ultimately expected.

When?

Disclosure of medical errors and adverse outcomes should occur as soon as it is apparent. Do not wait for a full understanding of circumstances before disclosure. This mistake will ultimately harm the relationship with the patient. It is far better to disclose that an error may have occurred, that an investigation is underway, and that the patient will be promptly informed of new information. If the provider involved in the event is unable to disclose immediately, their designee should step in to initiate discussion. Disclosure is often composed of a series of conversations over time. It is best to schedule disclosure conferences with the patient and family rather than to present the information without warning. The patient and/or the family should also have the contact information for a senior member of the team so that they can check on the progress of the investigation. They should also be given a general timeline for a complete analysis of the incident. It is helpful for the family to designate one person as the key contact for them to receive ongoing information.

Where?

Disclosure should occur in a setting appropriate for any serious clinical discussion. It is best to sit down at eye level with patients and minimize possible distractions. During inpatient care, disclosure may occur in a hospital room or consultation room, behind closed doors. Disclosures of events in the ambulatory setting may occur in a consultation room or the provider's office. It is not appropriate to perform disclosure in an executive suite. Disclosure of less serious events may be appropriate over the telephone. Providers should recognize that disclosure conversations may be recorded with audio or video devices. This type of activity should be permitted. Insisting that a disclosure conversation not be recorded is antithetical to the concept of transparency.

How?

The goals of the provider are to be empathetic and honest, without assigning blame. Clinical risk management professionals should be contacted to rehearse disclosure of serious errors whenever possible. The disclosure process is quite simple, although implementation may be emotionally difficult. It should begin with a description of the purpose of the conversation. In some circumstances it may be appropriate to follow the introduction of the conversation with an open-ended question about how much is understood about the event. In other circumstances it may be appropriate to begin by explaining the known facts. When the adverse event occurs during a procedure, consider referring back to the informed consent process.

It is recommended to explain the error or adverse event early in the conversation, in a way that is easily understood. Explain only what is known at the time, and that further information will be shared with the patient/family once it becomes available. It is important to avoid assigning blame or to discuss causes of the error at the initial disclosure. Initial understanding of the circumstances of the error is usually incomplete. Follow the description of the error with an explanation of what should have happened. Finally, review the potential consequences and the plan for ongoing treatment. An apology may be appropriate.

Disclosing providers should be prepared for the most common questions that occur:

- "How did this happen?"
- "How could you let this happen?"
- "I thought you said that this was safe?"

General responses to these types of questions are often best because the causes of the event may not be understood until a root-cause analysis is completed. Providers may respond that "we do not have the answers to all of these questions at this time, but we will be seeking to understand the event over the coming weeks." It is important to avoid assigning blame, even when one thinks that provider error is at the root cause. For example, in the case study of the magnesium sulfate medication error, a labeling error or a pump error may have contributed to the harm.

Finally, serious events that resulted in harm should be discussed with clinical risk management professionals before disclosure. There is immense value in rehearsing disclosure conversations. Most physicians are unprepared to respond to direct questions and accusations from grieving patients and family members.

IF YOU ARE SORRY—APOLOGIZE!

True friends stab you in the front.

—Oscar Wilde

While empathy is always appropriate when performing a disclosure, under certain circumstances it may also be appropriate to offer an apology. The goal of an apology is not to reduce to litigation but to maintain and restore trust between the provider and the patient. First and foremost the provider must feel that an apology is necessary. It is not recommended to apologize when the provider genuinely does not feel sorry for the occurrence. Neither the patient nor the provider will benefit from a forced and insincere apology. There is evidence that an apology may help providers to heal by diminishing their sense of guilt or shame.[18] An apology is also warranted when the event is inexcusable and indefensible—for example, removing the wrong limb in surgery. More

Box 1
States with "apology laws"

Arizona
California
Colorado
Connecticut
Delaware
Florida
Georgia
Hawaii
Idaho
Iowa
Indiana
Louisiana
Maine
Maryland
Massachusetts
Michigan
Missouri
Montana
Nebraska
New Hampshire
New Jersey
North Carolina
North Dakota
Ohio
Oklahoma
Oregon
South Carolina
South Dakota
Tennessee
Texas
Utah
Vermont
Virginia
Washington
West Virginia
Wyoming

commonly, events are complex and the provider may initially consider it appropriate to offer a more general apology In those circumstances, simply remarking that "we will keep you informed as more information becomes available—I am sorry" is recommended. The goal at that point is to not qualify or explain the apology, and to await the response.

Thirty-six states have "apology laws" that provide varying degrees of legal protection for apologies (**Box 1**). Generally these laws attempt to protect an apology from being admitted into court proceedings as an admission of guilt. Some states also provide similar protection for acts of benevolence such as writing off bills and hotel stays. The authors recommend discussing "apology laws" with your clinical risk management professional. There is contradictory evidence concerning whether apology laws alone have reduced or increased medical malpractice claims.[19,20]

EARLY RESOLUTION

The University of Michigan reported a reduction in medical malpractice expenditures after adopting a program between 2001 and 2007 to provide quick and fair compensation when appropriate. Most of these cases were identified before a lawsuit was ever filed. Early resolution of medical errors was paired with vigorous defense of cases in which care was appropriate. Numerous other large health systems have followed suit and are reporting similar reductions in malpractice expenditures. Adopting a formal program for early resolution most be approached systematically and comprehensively.[16]

Offering an apology for a serious safety event that resulted in harm without offering a mechanism for financially restoring the patient may explain the finding of increases in medical malpractice in some circumstances when an apology is offered.[19]

It may be helpful to think of this in terms of errors outside of the medical setting. If a contractor breaks something in your house during the course of performing repairs and discloses the event, offers a sincere apology, but makes no effort to restore you financially, there may be a higher likelihood of litigation.

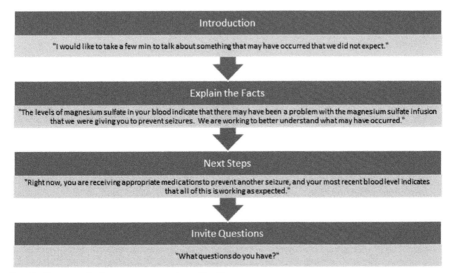

Fig. 1. How to disclose a suspected medication error.

SUMMARY

Disclosure of medical errors and adverse outcomes is expected by regulatory agencies and society as a whole. Providers are encouraged to seek training for disclosure and to seek professional help from Clinical Risk Management in disclosing any serious safety event that resulted in harm.

Recalling the unfortunate eclamptic patient in the case study, the treating physician should disclose the suspected medication error whenever the patient and family are available (**Fig. 1**). In this circumstance, the root causes were unknown. Therefore, a general comment stating that the magnesium sulfate level was found to be unexpectedly low. Why it was so low is unknown but will be fully investigated. Any new information will be promptly shared with the family. Irrespective of this problem, the providers will ensure that the mother and infant get the very best treatment. It would then be appropriate to ensure that appropriate treatment is being rendered currently, and that they will be kept informed as more information becomes available.

REFERENCES

1. Boothman RC. CANDOR: the antidote to deny and defend? Health Serv Res 2016;51:2487–90.
2. Golann D. Dropped medical malpractice claims: their surprising frequency, apparent causes, and potential remedies. Health Aff (Millwood) 2011;30: 1343–50.
3. Institute of Medicine. To err is human: building a safer health system. Committee on Quality of Health Care in America. Washington, DC: National Academy Press; 1999.
4. National Patient Safety Foundation. Free from harm: accelerating patient safety improvement fifteen years after to err is human. Boston: National Patient Safety Foundation; 2015.
5. Martin MA, Daniel M. Medical error—the third leading cause of death in the US. BMJ 2016;353:i2139.
6. Joint Commission on Accreditation of Healthcare Organizations. Comprehensive accreditation manual for hospitals: the official handbook. Oakbrook Terrace (IL): Joint Commission on Accreditation of Healthcare Organizations; 2001. p. RI. 1.2.2.
7. National health expenditure data, historical. Available at: https://www.cms.gov/ Research-Statistics-Data-and-Systems/Statistics-Trends-and-Reports/National HealthExpendData/NationalHealthAccountsHistorical.html. Accessed September 28, 2018.
8. Website Claxton G, Rae M, Levitt L, et al. How have healthcare prices grown in the U.S. over time?. Available at: https://www.healthsystemtracker.org/chart-collection/how-have-healthcare-prices-grown-in-the-u-s-over-time/. Accessed September 28, 2018.
9. Council on Ethical and Judicial Affairs. In: Code of medical ethics of the American Medical Association: current opinions with annotations. 2008-2009. Chicago: American Medical Association; 2009.
10. Witman AB, Park DM, Hardin SB. How do patients want physicians to handle mistakes? A survey of internal medicine patients in an academic setting. Arch Intern Med 1996;156:2565–9.
11. Holden RJ, Karsh BT. A review of medical error reporting system design considerations and proposed cross-level systems research framework: human factors. Hum Factors 2007;49(2):257–76.

12. Barach P, Small SD. Reporting and preventing medical mishaps: lessons from non-medical near miss reporting systems. BMJ 2000;320(7237):759–63.
13. Kaldjian LC, Jones EW, We BJ, et al. Reporting medical errors to improve patient safety: a survey of physicians in teaching hospitals. Arch Intern Med 2008;168: 40–6.
14. Ricci M, Goldman AP, de Leval MR, et al. Pitfalls of adverse event reporting in pediatric cardiac intensive care. Arch Dis Child 2004;89:856–9.
15. Liang BA. A system of medical error disclosure. Qual Saf Health Care 2002;11(1): 64–8.
16. Boothman R, Imhoff SJ, Campbell DA. Nurturing a culture of patient safety and achieving lower malpractice risk through disclosure: lessons learned and future directions. Front Health Serv Manage 2012;28(3):13–27.
17. The Joint Commission. Hospital Accreditation Standards. TJC RI.01.02.01. Oak Brook (IL): Department of Publications and Education, Joint Commission Resources; 2017.
18. Leape L. Full disclosure and apology—an idea whose time has come. Physician Exec 2006;32(2):16–8.
19. McMichael BJ, Van Horn R, Kip Viscusi W. Sorry is never enough: how state apology laws fail to reduce medical malpractice liability risk. Stanford Law Review, Forthcoming. Available at SSRN: https://papers.ssrn.com/sol3/papers.cfm?abstract_id=2883693. Accessed February 27, 2019.
20. Weber DO. "Who's sorry now?". Physician Exec 2006;6:11–4.

Role of Patient Safety Organizations in Improving Patient Safety

Jason Boulanger, MFA[a],[*],[1], Carol Keohane, MS, BSN, RN[a],[2], Ashley Yeats, MD[b],[3]

KEYWORDS

- Patient safety organization (PSO) • Patient safety evaluation system (PSES)
- Patient safety and quality improvement act (PSQIA) • Privilege • Confidentiality
- Peer review

KEY POINTS

- A culture of safety, specifically one that continuously learns from error, is essential to effective and safe obstetric and gynecologic care.
- Reporting, analysis, measurement of, and the deliberation of health care professionals with subject-matter expertise on health care–associated errors are critical to a culture of continuous learning and safety.
- Learning from errors requires transparency, commitment, and open dialogue, so that factors contributing to patient harm can be examined in an honest manner.
- Membership in a Patient Safety Organization provides an opportunity for providers across the spectrum of health care to leverage confidentiality and privilege from the federal government in order to reduce the anxiety of litigation or other actions that limit providers' willingness to report errors.

A learning organization is one that is successful at acquiring, cultivating, and applying knowledge that can be used to help it continually adapt to change.[1]

The Institute of Medicine's (IOM) "To Err Is Human"[2] report published in 1999 asserted that medical errors were responsible for between 44,000 and 98,000 deaths annually in American hospitals, serving as a call to action for the patient safety community to improve care delivery.

Disclosure Statement: The authors have no disclosures to make.
[a] Patient Safety, CRICO/RMF, 1325 Boylston Street, Boston, MA 02215, USA; [b] Beth Israel Deaconess Hospital–Milton, 199 Reedsdale Road, Milton, MA 02186, USA
[1] Lead author.
[2] Senior author.
[3] Coauthor.
* Corresponding author.
E-mail address: jboulanger@rmf.harvard.edu

Obstet Gynecol Clin N Am 46 (2019) 257–267
https://doi.org/10.1016/j.ogc.2019.02.001
0889-8545/19/© 2019 Elsevier Inc. All rights reserved.

Research into the incidence of harm and death resulting from medical error continued after this landmark report. One study argued that the reported prevalence of medical error–related death in the IOM report was grossly underestimated and that the incidence was likely greater than 200,000 deaths per year.[3] Debate of the actual incidence of harm from medical errors continues, but most patient safety experts would agree that medical errors still occur at considerable and unacceptable rates.

These estimates create an urgent need for the continued attention and examination of medical errors. Patient Safety Organizations (PSO) are a federal program that enables providers across the health care delivery system to learn from errors, analyze those errors at both system and discrete case levels, identify factors in those errors that ultimately led to patient harm, design, and implement risk mitigation interventions, and to do so with the protection of privilege and confidentiality.

A culture of safety, specifically one that continuously learns from error, is essential to effective and safe obstetric and gynecologic care. Reporting, analysis, measurement of, and the deliberation of health care professionals with subject-matter expertise on health care–associated errors are critical to a culture of continuous learning and safety. Learning from errors requires transparency, commitment, and open dialogue, so that factors contributing to patient harm can be examined in an honest manner.

The IOM report also expressed the need for "voluntary reporting systems [to] provide an important complement to the mandatory system" and that "Congress should enact laws to protect the confidentiality of certain information collected."[2] Membership in a PSO provides an opportunity for providers across the spectrum of health care to leverage confidentiality and privilege from the federal government in order to reduce the anxiety of litigation or other actions that limit providers' willingness to report errors. As Dr. Daniel Ofri notes, "As doctors, if we fail, it's not something outside of us; it *is* us. We are the error. The shame is so powerful that most doctors will never come forward about an error."[4] The emotional impact of both error and harm underscores the value of anonymity, confidentiality, and privilege to the learning process. Without those protections, the barriers to enhancing a culture of safety and establishing a learning environment would be insurmountable. Furthermore, the ability to deliberate on the causes of medical error in a protected environment allows for greater transparency and likely reduces the shame associated with the admission and reporting of a provider's own medical error. In addition to articulating the need for a system of voluntary and confidential reporting, the IOM's report went on to state that legislation establishing privilege and confidentiality would be necessary, as "without such legislation, health care organizations and providers may be discouraged from participating."[2]

PSOs offer an opportunity to aggregate data across large health care delivery systems, hospitals, and practice groups. "Regardless of the practice setting—whether employed by a hospital, in a large multispecialty group, or remaining in independent practice—all physicians will have to change some aspects of their behavior. Relevant and meaningful change can only occur based on measured performance. Measured performance produces data about what needs to be improved. By definition then, the collection of these data provides a threshold statement of suboptimal performance."[5] The aggregation of data from many providers makes that "threshold statement of suboptimal performance" more accurate and stronger.

In 2005, following the publication, "To Err Is Human," and the public's response, Congress passed the Patient Safety and Quality Improvement Act (PSQIA), which afforded health care providers with privilege and confidentiality protections in an effort to "encourage organizations to identify errors, evaluate causes and design systems to prevent future errors from occurring."[6]

The PSQIA is a necessary adjunct to the Health Care Quality Improvement Act (HCQIA), which was silent on the privilege of peer review materials.[7] As Gosfield[7] relates, at least one court, in a decision, stated that the "HCQIA [was] no longer Congress's final word on the issue of medical peer review, acknowledging that the PSQIA was enacted with the intent to encourage a culture of safety by providing for broad confidentiality and legal protections."

Acknowledging that existing state-level peer review protections were inconsistent, ineffective, and only covered hospital-based care, the PSQIA established "uniform, federal standards for confidentiality of information about patient safety events."[8] On January 19, 2009, the Executive Office of Health and Human Services issued the Patient Safety Rule,[9] which defined the data and information that are collected with and for the benefit of privilege and confidentiality, that is, Patient Safety Work Product (PSWP), the processes and systems by which PSWP is collected, aggregated, and analyzed, that is, the Patient Safety Evaluation System (PSES), and the federal offices and agencies that oversee Patient Safety Activities and impose fines, that is, the Agency for Healthcare Research and Quality (AHRQ) and the Office of Civil Rights (OCR).

"The PSO itself is a private entity subject to regulations and administration by AHRQ."[5] PSOs are not federally funded. They operate pursuant to private contracts with providers reporting to them. Providers contract with a PSO to receive and analyze PSWP they submit. To qualify as a "listed" organization, a PSO must meet standards that are set forth in the federal regulations.[8] Certain types of entities are prohibited from applying or acting: health insurance companies, a unit or division of a health insurer, an entity that is managed or controlled by a health insurer. In addition, the Act also disqualifies public or private entities with statutory or regulatory authority over health providers (eg, accreditation and licensure bodies) from seeking listing as a PSO.

Implementation of the Patient Safety Rule of the PSQIA established 8 required patient safety activities of AHRQ-listed PSOs:

1. Efforts to improve patient safety and the quality of health care delivery;
2. The collection and analysis of patient safety work product;
3. The development and dissemination of information with respect to improving patient safety, such as recommendations, protocols, or information regarding best practices;
4. The utilization of patient safety work product for the purposes of encouraging a culture of safety and of providing feedback and assistance to effectively minimize patient risk;
5. The maintenance of procedures to preserve confidentiality with respect to patient safety work product;
6. The provision of appropriate security measures with respect to patient safety work product;
7. The utilization of qualified staff; and
8. Activities related to the operation of a patient safety evaluation system and to the provision of feedback to participants in a patient safety evaluation system.[9]

The final rule also provided a formal definition for PSWP, the information for which privilege and confidentiality may be applied. It is defined as "data which could improve patient safety, health care quality, or health care outcomes." In addition, data for which an organization wishes to apply the term "PSWP" (and the subsequent privilege and confidentiality) must be assembled or developed for reporting to a PSO and be reported to a PSO.[9] PSWP may include both provider and patient information. Analysis is an important feature.

As AHRQ states, "The Patient Safety Rule relies primarily upon a system of attestations, which places a significant burden for understanding and complying with these requirements on the PSO."[10] However, the Patient Safety Rule also authorizes AHRQ to conduct reviews (including announced or unannounced site visits) to assess PSO compliance. To assist PSOs in making the required attestations and preparing for a compliance review, AHRQ developed "Patient Safety Organizations: A Compliance Self-Assessment Guide to suggest approaches for thinking systematically about the scope of these requirements and what compliance may mean for an individual PSO."[10]

AHRQ, one of 11 agencies within the federal government's Department of Health and Human Services and the lead federal agency for patient safety research, is charged with overseeing the implementation of the PSQIA and administering the PSO program. Administration of the program includes oversight of the certification processes for listing and delisting, verifying (through audits) that PSOs meet their obligations under the Patient Safety Rule, working with PSOs to correct any deficiencies in the operations, and, if necessary, revoking the listing of a PSO that remains out of compliance with the requirements. AHRQ also retains responsibility for developing, maintaining, and updating the Common Formats, a set of common definitions that facilitate the collection, reporting, aggregation, and analysis of patient safety events. That aggregation is done within the Network of Patient Safety Databases, to which PSOs submit relevant, unidentifiable patient safety error data.

The OCR is responsible for the investigation and enforcement of the confidentiality provisions defined through the Patient Safety Rule. As noted, "OCR will investigate allegations of violations of confidentiality through a complaint-driven system. To the extent practicable, OCR will seek cooperation in obtaining compliance with the confidentiality provisions, including providing technical assistance. When OCR is unable to achieve an informal resolution of an indicated violation through voluntary compliance, the HHS Secretary has the discretion to impose a civil money penalty of up to $11,000 against any PSO, provider, or responsible person for each *knowing and reckless* disclosure that is in violation of the confidentiality provisions."[11] It is important that all providers participating in PSO activities are educated and understand the rules governing the confidentiality protections that apply to designated patient safety work product (PSWP). The confidentiality provisions and federal privilege continue to apply to information deemed PSWP, even in instances of a violation.[11]

Although the Department of Health and Human Services published the Final Rule in 2009, the federal government in 2010 further outlined requirements in the Patient Protection and Affordable Care Act (ACA), which includes a requirement that hospitals with a high readmission rate and those of more than 50 beds who seek to provide care for a qualified health plan through the exchanges under health reform be "required to have a Patient Safety Evaluation system, which means a relationship [contract] with a PSO."[12] The requirement was phased in and is thought to have increased PSO utilization.[13] Although the ACA's mandate provides a valuable incentive for certain hospitals to participate, it should be noted that a qualified health plan may also contract with a "health care provider if that provider implements such mechanisms to improve health care quality as the Secretary may by regulation require."[14] Other methods by which a provider may satisfy this requirement include participation in a Health Enterprise Network or having a contract with a Quality Improvement Organization.[15]

AHRQ first implemented the PSO program with a vision to create a national repository of patient safety error reports. The assumption was that the privilege and confidentiality that the Patient Safety Act affords would reduce the anxiety associated with error reporting and increase the number of event reports submitted to that database. The database, therefore, would represent a more accurate picture of patient safety errors and associated outcomes in the United States. The value of a representative sample of national patient safety errors cannot be understated. In collaboration with the Federal Patient Safety Workgroup, the National Quality Forum, and the public, AHRQ has developed Common Formats, containing structured definitions and a taxonomy for categorizing patient safety errors related to acute care hospitals and skilled nursing facilities. Most recently, AHRQ released Common Formats for Surveillance — Hospital to gather information through retrospective review of medical records as a complementary aid for the detection and calculation of adverse events beyond traditional reporting mechanisms.[16] Despite these coordinated efforts, the development and adoption of the Common Formats have been challenging. Data submissions to the National Patient Safety Database (NPSD) have been limited. Only 30% of the known error reporting held by PSOs has been reported to the NPSD.[17] A recent educational brief aimed at assisting PSOs in implementing the AHRQ Common Formats for patient safety reporting by health care providers highlights some of the challenges associated with the use of the Common Formats and submission process. For example, interviews with key stakeholders, including several PSOs, revealed the following suggestions to increase the ease of implementation: "AHRQ Common Formats should reflect workflow, and provide more detail on factors contributing to safety events."[17] In addition, the report notes that "AHRQ should continue to provide transparency into future plans for development of the AHRQ Common Formats."[17]

Despite the slow pace of error report submissions, PSOs have harvested unique opportunities to leverage the privilege and confidentiality through safe table convenings, a privileged and confidential forum in which providers may collectively analyze error report. Those forums have engendered robust, transparent dialogue among a broad diversity of clinicians.

In parallel, there have been several instances whereby the privilege and confidentiality of the PSQIA have been challenged in the court system. These recent instances of case law have provided clarity on how an organization should conduct their patient safety activities in order to maintain that privilege and how the federal law interacts with state-level legislation and regulation.

Relevant case law has sought to clarify both the relationship between state and federal laws and the extent to which the privilege and confidentiality afforded by the PSQIA may be applied. Two recent examples of case law provide relevant points of reference, even though the depth of case law on the PSQIA is shallow. In *Department of Financial and Professional Regulation v. Walgreen Co.*, the Appellate Court upheld the designation of incident reports as privileged PSWP because the defendant, Walgreens, submitted affidavits demonstrating that the requested incident reports were collected in a "Strategic Reporting and Analytical Reporting System that was a defined component of Walgreen's PSES." This ruling underscores the importance of accurately describing the components of a PSO participant's PSES.[18] In addition, in *Tibbs v. Bunnell*, in which the Supreme Court of Kentucky compelled the release of PSWP, the PSQIA "was not be construed to limit a provider's recordkeeping obligations under federal, state, or local law."[19] Although a strong dissenting opinion was put forth in the Supreme Court of Kentucky's decision, this outcome also emphasizes that thorough documentation of a PSES, rigor in how analysis is conducted within a PSES, and the ultimate reporting of PSWP to a PSO is instrumental to the maintenance of privilege.

THE ROAD AHEAD IN RESPONSE TO CHANGING HEALTH CARE DELIVERY

PSOs are in a unique position to improve care delivery by fostering cross-collaboration in quality and safety between hospitals, provider groups, and other designated health care providers. Opportunities exist to leverage the PSO to create learning collaboratives among multiple providers. The extension of federal peer review protections beyond the inpatient setting allows for the investigation and analysis of care delivery across a continuum of care that includes care provided in ambulatory and long-term care settings.

Authorized by the ACA and effective with inpatient hospital discharges beginning October 1, 2012, the Centers for Medicare and Medicaid Services (CMS) established hospital payment incentive programs, including the Hospital *Value-Based Purchasing* (VBP) Program and Hospital *Readmissions Reduction Program* (HRRP). The structure of the VPB program, as described by CMS, financially rewards hospitals based on the following:

- The quality of care provided to Medicare patients
- How closely best clinical practices are followed
- How well hospitals enhance patients' experiences of care during hospital stays[20]

The stated intent of the HRRP program is to "make Americans' health care better by linking payment to the quality of hospital care. It gives hospitals a strong financial incentive to:

- Make their communication and care coordination efforts better;
- Work better with patients and caregivers on postdischarge planning."[20]

Payment incentive programs, also adopted and adapted by other payers and accrediting agencies, mark a transition in the changing health care environment from remuneration for volume-based care to remuneration for value-based care. The creation of Affordable Care Organizations and the extension of payer "payment risk contracts" to provider groups have placed the individual provider income at risk, aligning incentives for providers, hospitals, and health care delivery systems to engage in joint initiatives to improve quality and safety.

Driven by concern for nonsustainable increases in US health care delivery costs and supported by imperatives, such as the Institute for Healthcare Improvement's *The Triple Aim* (improving patient experience of care, improving the health of populations, reducing per capita cost of health care)[21] as well as (i) improving quality and safety; (ii) heightening focus on risk mitigation; (iii) adapting high reliability organization principles[22]; and (iv) coordinating transitions of care, presents challenges for health care providers and organizations and opportunities for PSOs.

In addition, changes in reimbursement structures (ie, the 2018 Outpatient Prospective Payment System Final Rule, in which CMS removed total knee replacement from the Medicare inpatient-only list) will continue to influence the shift in care delivery from the inpatient to ambulatory environment. Not only do reimbursement structures influence the increasing use of outpatient procedures, but also some experts believe that several gynecologic procedures are well suited to the ambulatory setting. Endometrial ablations, hysteroscopy, bladder neck extension, reconstruction of the pelvic floor, sterilization, procedures for uterine bleeding, fibroids, ovarian cysts, and D&Cs (dilation and curettage) are examples of high-throughput procedures that can be performed in the ambulatory surgical center (ASC).[23] Assessing and monitoring quality and safety in areas such as ASCs, procedural areas, and ambulatory clinics will be an important progression toward evaluating patient safety in the evolving landscape of health care delivery.

Patient Safety Organizations and the Changing Health Care Delivery Environment

There are currently 85 PSOs listed by AHRQ.[24] The structure, function, purpose, and communities served by these various PSOs vary, but are unified by an overarching mission of improving patient safety. The authors' experience of the value of PSOs in the changing health care delivery environment highlights the value of PSO membership.

Root cause analysis

Through PSO membership, member organizations submit as PSWP to the PSO actual root cause analysis (RCA) summary, learnings, and contributing factors related to adverse events that have occurred within their organization. Action items from similar adverse events occurring at other member organizations may be provided by the PSO to the submitting organization upon request.

The robust submission of RCA PSWP across a synergistic membership provides a rich database of patient safety events that is curated by the PSO and analyzed within the PSO's PSES for emerging patient safety trends. The Michigan Health and Hospital Association (MHA) Keystone Center PSO has elected to address birth-related adverse events that "lead to severe injury or death, including severe bleeding, infections, and high blood pressure."[25] The MHA Keystone Center has identified that communication issues and a lack of standardized protocols lead to adverse obstetric events.[25] Patient Safety Alerts, that incorporate information that is rendered contextually nonidentifiable by the PSO, not only raises awareness of key areas of risk but also promulgates lessons learned and best practices across the PSO membership.

Areas of emerging risk and/or patterns of harm events identified across member institutions serve as a signal to convene multidisciplinary "safe table" convenings of key stakeholders from PSO member organizations. A safe table serves as a forum for debriefing and may be initiated by the PSO at the behest of its membership or requested by a member organization.

Safe table convenings

Safe table convenings, hosted by a PSO within the construct of the PSO's PSES, provide a protected forum for discussion and analysis of shared patient safety concerns, with federal privilege and confidentiality provisions afforded by the PSQIA. Information discussed in the safe table forum (PSWP) is governed by the PSQIA and is not discoverable, nor subject to subpoena. The environment is akin to the peer review environment that exists in some states. However, protections extend beyond a hospital's traditional peer review structure. It may also include a broader definition of health care provider (eg, Emergency Medical Service [EMS] providers, retail pharmacy, private practice physician group) than is traditionally described in medical staff bylaws or recognized under state law.

With the privilege of federally conferred confidentiality provisions comes a personal responsibility or "burden" not to disclose the information shared (PSWP) during a safe table, including the potential for a personal fine of $11,000.[11]

This "safe" environment fosters rich, robust discussion and sharing of knowledge from which a PSO may generate best practice guidelines and risk mitigation strategies informed by the engagement of frontline providers and subject matter experts. Examples include The Academic Medical Center PSO's neonatal encephalopathy guidelines, "Therapeutic Hypothermia in Neonates," which were based on the collective literature review and deliberations of "subject matter experts in Neonatology, Neurology, Maternal Fetal Medicine, Obstetrics and Gynecology, and Pediatrics."[26] The Quality Center Patient Safety Organization in North Carolina engaged in an opioid stewardship effort that resulted in the North Carolina Guidelines for Pain Management in the Emergency Department, a 13-point guide to best practices to reduce opioid overprescribing through opioid prescription limitations, use of non-opioid medications, and consulting the North Carolina Controlled Substances Reporting System.[27] The Academic Medical Center Patient Safety Organization released Patient Safety Guidance for Electronic Health Record Downtime, which serves as a complementary tool to hospitals' emergency management systems in providing a "patient safety lens" to electronic health record (EHR) Downtime risks. The publication highlights patient safety priorities, such as downtime alerts and notifications, activating a command center and operations, communication and messaging strategies, and planning for recovery and deactivation. The guidance document serves as a playbook that includes an action plan checklist to assist hospitals during periods of extended EHR Downtime.[28] Another novel approach afforded through participation in a PSO can be seen through the work of The Center for Patient Safety (CPS) PSO, which focuses on learning and understanding medical errors that occur during EMS care, why they occur, and how to prevent patient harm. The CPS PSO, which contracts with EMS providers, has steadily seen its membership grow since its listing in 2011. This growth is seen as a reflection of the value participation brings to understanding patient safety within EMS.[27]

A PSO may engage in the socialization and dissemination of consensus guidelines across its membership, a process facilitated by having key organizational stakeholders and leaders involved in the safe table, which may involve a series of safe stable forums spanning several months.

The shared learning garnered from PSO-curated RCAs and participation in PSO-hosted safe table forums provide opportunities for health care providers and organizations to improve care in the rapidly changing health care delivery paradigm described above.

The role of patient safety organizations in response to mergers and acquisitions: creating a system view of quality and safety

Member organizations of a PSO interact with a PSO through their own PSES. A member organization's PSES is designed and maintained for the collection, management, or analysis of information for reporting to or by a PSO. Resources are available online from organizations such as the Alliance for Quality Improvement and Patient Safety.[29]

Driven by market forces and consumer demand for improved access to health care, integration of hospitals and provider groups into merged health systems continues to transform care delivery. Coordination of care across care transitions, via disparate EHRs, and related to transfer of patients between affiliated entities poses unique patient safety challenges. Peer review, if supported by state statute, may not extend across hospital licenses, limiting robust peer review at a network level.

PSO membership provides opportunity to advance a health system's quality and safety agenda at the network level. System level patient safety improvement has become increasingly relevant in the current market environment of hospital and provider organization mergers and acquisitions.

An emerging area of interest in the PSO community, and an opportunity for health systems, is the concept of a PSO enterprise agreement, in which a health system enters into "enterprise agreement" with a PSO. The enterprise agreement in turn facilitates the creation of a health system "enterprise PSES" (**Fig. 1**) that encompasses the individual PSESs of its "owned" hospitals and provider groups.[30]

An enterprise PSES may afford a unique opportunity for networked hospitals and provider groups to share internally, certain patient safety activities, peer review activities, and RCAs across their hospital licenses and medical staffs. An enterprise PSES thus supports mechanisms to internally align best practices and to improve patient outcomes at a system or network level. It should be noted that, to date, there is a

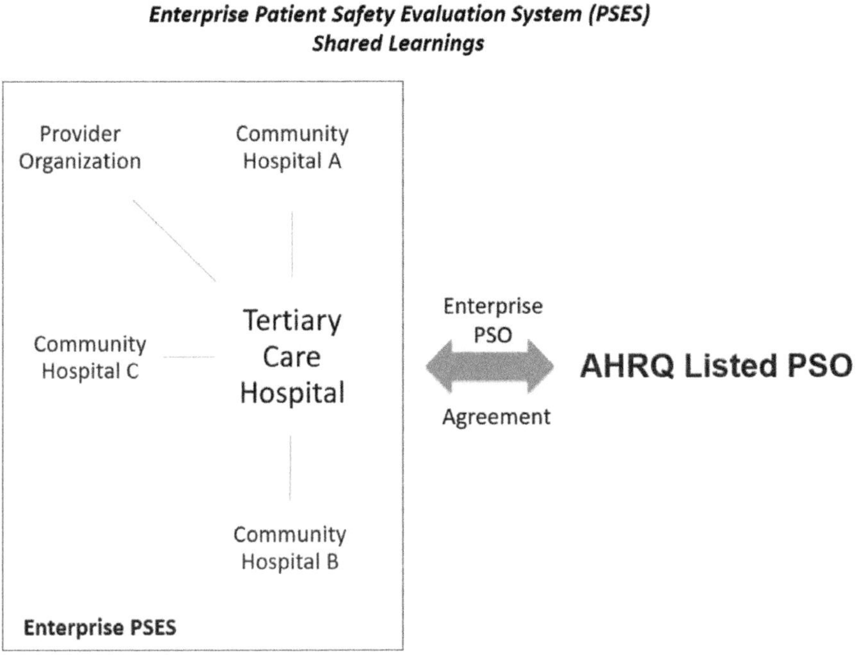

Enterprise Patient Safety Evaluation System (PSES)
Shared Learnings

Fig. 1. Select care reviews via reporting/analysis pathway by individual institutions for global tracking/trending and identification of emerging risks.

paucity of case law relative to the assertion of privilege presumed to be applied to the analysis and deliberations of patient safety activities within an enterprise PSES.

In conclusion, health care delivery organizations have a unique opportunity to advance efforts to improve patient safety through participation in PSOs. PSO programs provide a forum for understanding, collaboration, and translation of evidence into practice at a faster pace than traditional methods of scientific review and deliberation. Perhaps most importantly, PSO programs help to promote a culture of safety in support of medicine's primary tenet to *"primum non nocere,"* first, do no harm.

REFERENCES

1. Dotan DB. Patient safety organizations. J Clin Eng 2009;34(3):142–6.
2. Institute of Medicine (US) Committee on quality of health care in America. 2, Errors in health care: a leading cause of death and Injury. In: Kohn LT, Corrigan JM, Donaldson MS, editors. To err is human: building a safer health system. Washington (DC): National Academies Press (US); 2000. Available from: https://www.ncbi.nlm.nih.gov/books/NBK225187/.
3. Makary MA, Daniel M. Medical error—the third leading cause of death in the US. BMJ 2016;353:i2139.
4. Greenberg R. The dirty secret about medical errors. 2017. The Huffington Post. Available at: https://www.huffingtonpost.com/riva-greenberg/medical-errors_b_3535171.html. Accessed September 25, 2018.
5. Using patient safety organizations to further clinical integration. Available at: https://www.gosfield.com/images/PDF/Greenbranch.MPM.Using_PSOs_to_Further_CI.MarApr_2014.pdf. Accessed September 25, 2018.

6. United States Congress. Patient safety and quality improvement act of 2005. Washington, DC: U.S. G.P.O.; 2005.

7. Gosfield A. Five reasons physicians should use patient safety organizations. Arlington (VA): Bloomberg Law; 2014.

8. Clancy CM. Patient safety organizations ready for action. AORN J 2009;89(2): 385–7.

9. US Department of Health and Human Services. Patient Safety Rule. 73 FR 70796. Available at: https://www.ecfr.gov/cgi-bin/text-idx?SID=42192f8b6c83ddc436 beeab06ef0ab90&mc=true&node=pt42.1.3&rgn=div5. Accessed September 26, 2018.

10. Patient safety organizations: a compliance self-assessment guide. Available at: https://www.pso.ahrq.gov/sites/default/files/wysiwyg/saguide.pdf. Accessed October 1, 2018.

11. HHS Office of the Secretary Office for Civil Rights, OCR. Confidentiality provisions of the patient safety act. HHS.gov; 2017. Available at: https://www.hhs.gov/hipaa/ for-professionals/patient-safety/enforcement/index.html. Accessed September 27, 2018.

12. ACA PSO mandate. CHPSO. Available at: http://www.chpso.org/post/aca-pso-mandate. Accessed September 26, 2018.

13. Munier WB, Cousins D. The changing PSO landscape: national perspective 2015. Available at: https://www.centerforpatientsafety.org/2015/06/30/the-changing-pso-landscape-national-legal-perspectives/.

14. Compilation of Patient Protection and Affordable Care Act: as Amended through November 1, 2010 Including Patient Protection and Affordable Care Act Health-Related Portions of the Health Care and Education Reconciliation Act of 2010; 2010.

15. Callahan M, Flynn E, Pavkovic S. PSO 101: overview of patient safety act 2016. Available at: https://www.kattenlaw.com/pso-101-overview-of-patient-safety-act.

16. Frequently asked questions. AHRQ. Available at: https://pso.ahrq.gov/faq. Accessed October 1, 2018.

17. Lessons From PSOs on Applying the AHRQ Common Formats for …. Available at: https://pso.ahrq.gov/sites/default/files/wysiwyg/npsd-common-formats-brief.pdf. Accessed September 26, 2018.

18. Binzer P. PSQIA cases. Alliance for quality improvement and patient safety. Available at: http://www.allianceforqualityimprovement.org/psqia-cases. Accessed September 27, 2018.

19. Airapetian Z. Federal privilege under patient and quality improvement act: the impact of Tibbs v. Bunell. J Health Biomed Law 2016;11:345–89.

20. Hospital value-based purchasing. Available at: https://www.cms.gov/Outreach-and-Education/Medicare-Learning-Network-MLN/MLNProducts/downloads/ Hospital_VBPurchasing_Fact_Sheet_ICN907664.pdf. Accessed September 27, 2018.

21. The IHI triple aim. Institute for Healthcare Improvement. Available at: http://www. ihi.org/Engage/Initiatives/TripleAim/Pages/default.aspx. Accessed September 27, 2018.

22. CRICO. Available at: https://www.rmf.harvard.edu/Clinician-Resources/Article/ 2017/White-Paper-Safety-Culture-and-Risk-Reliability-in-Health-Care. Accessed September 27, 2018.

23. 5 things to know about Gynecology in ASCs. Available at: https://www. beckersasc.com/news-analysis/5-things-to-know-about-gynecology-in-ascs.html. Accessed October 24, 2018.

24. Federally-Listed PSOs. AHRQ. 2010. Available at: https://pso.ahrq.gov/listed. Accessed September 27, 2018.
25. MHA Keystone Center PSO Members Discuss Obstetrical Events at Safe Table. Available at: https://www.mha.org/Newsroom/ID/1503/MHA-Keystone-Center-PSO-Members-Discuss-Obstetrical-Events-at-Safe-Table. Accessed October 24, 2018.
26. Neonatal encephalopathy guidelines. Available at: https://www.rmf.harvard.edu/Clinician-Resources/Guidelines-Algorithms/2016/Neonatal-Encephalopathy. Accessed October 24, 2018.
27. Stories from the Field. AHRQ. Available at: https://pso.ahrq.gov/with_PSO/stories. Accessed September 27, 2018.
28. CRICO. Available at: https://www.rmf.harvard.edu/Clinician-Resources/Guidelines-Algorithms/2017/EHR-Downtime-Guidelines. Accessed September 27, 2018.
29. Binzer P. Resources. Alliance for quality improvement and patient safety. Available at: http://www.allianceforqualityimprovement.org/resources. Accessed September 27, 2018.
30. Sands K, Yeats A. Keynote – Innovation in Root Cause Analysis and PSES Structure, The Alliance for Quality Improvement and Patient Safety AQIPS Annual Patient Safety Organization and Provider Convention Legal and Litigation Conference, Washington, DC, September 17–18, 2017.

Implementation and Change Management

The Certification Process Driving Patient Safety

Pooja Shivraj, MS, PhD[a], Amanda Novak, MEd[b], Sylvia Aziz, MHA[b], Wilma Larsen, MD[c], Susan Ramin, MD[b],*

KEYWORDS

- Patient safety • Certification • Assessment • Learning • Practice

KEY POINTS

- The American Board of Obstetrics and Gynecology (ABOG) intentionally incorporates patient safety into its initial and continuous certification processes to drive the safe practice of medicine.
- Embedding patient safety within initial certification at ABOG includes, but is not limited to, assessing candidates' ability to diagnose conditions accurately and practice safe medicine.
- Integrating patient safety in continuous certification at ABOG also includes, but is not limited to, simulation experiences improving team communication and current technology enhancing diagnostic accuracy.
- It is hypothesized that learning and actively engaging in initial and continuous certification at ABOG that intentionally embeds patient safety would help diplomates practice safely.

INTRODUCTION

The American Board of Obstetrics and Gynecology (ABOG), a nonprofit organization that board certifies obstetricians and gynecologists, was founded in 1927 and incorporated in 1930. The ABOG also offers continuous certification (maintenance of certification [MOC]) to obstetricians and gynecologists in the United States and Canada. Board certification by the ABOG is a voluntary process for those physicians who choose to pursue and maintain their certification for the specialty of obstetrics and gynecology. In addition, ABOG offers subspecialty board certifications in female pelvic medicine and reconstructive surgery, gynecologic oncology, maternal-fetal medicine, and reproductive endocrinology and infertility.

Disclosure Statement: None of the authors have any conflicts of interest or financial ties to disclose.
[a] American Board of Obstetrics and Gynecology, 2915 Vine Street, Dallas, TX 75204, USA;
[b] Maintenance of Certification, American Board of Obstetrics and Gynecology, 2915 Vine Street, Dallas, TX 75204, USA; [c] Examinations, American Board of Obstetrics and Gynecology, 2915 Vine Street, Dallas, TX 75204, USA
* Corresponding author.
E-mail address: sramin@abog.org

The ABOG is one of the 24 member boards of the American Board of Medical Specialties (ABMS). The ABMS works to maintain standards for initial and continuous certification in order to improve the quality of health care to patients, families, and communities.[1] In 2016, the ABMS, in conjunction with the National Patient Safety Foundation (NPSF), issued a joint call encouraging each ABMS member board to integrate patient safety principles and activities into the initial and continuous certification.[2] The joint call for patient safety included, but were not limited to:

- Safe and effective diagnoses
- Diagnostic pitfalls
- Safety in the ambulatory care setting
- Engaging the team in diagnostic accuracy
- Engaging patients and families
- The role of health care information technology in diagnostic accuracy
- Simulation experiences that improve team communication
- Specialty considerations for diagnostic accuracy
- Medication safety

It was also determined that approved practice-relevant safety activities would integrate the core competencies, as defined by ABMS and the Accreditation Council for Graduate Medical Education (ACGME), while meeting the individual needs of the diplomates.[3] In the certification process that ABOG defines for its candidates and diplomates, patient safety is the bare minimum expectation upon which knowledge and skills build. Because diplomates are expected to understand patient safety principles within their specialties and subspecialties, they need to be evaluated appropriately within the certification process to ensure that they not only have an understanding of those safety principles but also maintain and implement them over time. The ABOG hence incorporates patient safety into both its initial and continuous certification (MOC) processes to ensure diplomates have sufficient knowledge of safety science and principles to practice safe medicine and diagnose patients correctly so their patients can expect both quality and safe care.

The purpose of this article is to describe how ABOG's initial and continuous certification processes integrate various aspects of patient safety principles to ensure as much as possible that diplomates practice safely. In the first section, the authors describe how the assessments within initial and continuous certification processes are integral in knowing and learning about patient safety.

The Theories of Knowing and Learning

Curriculum, instruction, and assessment play a pivotal role in learning and knowing, creating a reciprocal influence on each other.[4–9] Curriculum refers to the knowledge and skills that examinees are supposed to learn. Specific to patient safety within this article, curriculum refers to the expectation that ABOG holds for diplomates relevant to competence in quality improvement (QI) and patient safety. Instruction refers to activities conducted by the examinee and the instructor to help master the objectives specified by the curriculum. In relation to patient safety, instruction within this article refers to how the examinee learns the content specified by ABOG during his or her residency and fellowship (external instruction) and also how he or she learns the content while studying for examinations based on blueprint specifications (self-instruction). Finally, assessment is the method used to measure the outcome of achievement regarding the competencies of interest. With respect to patient safety within the context of this article, assessment refers to how well the examinee or diplomate has mastered content relating to patient safety to apply it to the field. Ideally, all 3 functions should be coordinated such that the assessment should measure the content of the curriculum that examinees are expected to master through instruction or learning. This inter-relationship is depicted in **Fig. 1**.[9] It is hypothesized that when patient safety is actively embedded in the content mandated within initial and continuous certification at ABOG, candidates and diplomates learn that content and then seek to actively implement it within their practice.

The Assessment Triangle: a Process of Reasoning from Evidence

Incorporating patient safety content in ABOG's assessments within both initial and continuous certification procedures serves as a process of reasoning from evidence.[9] ABOG cannot directly measure patient safety knowledge, skills, understanding or cognition of examinees or diplomates. However, the ABOG does create observational tools, such as certifying examinations that include low-fidelity simulation for malpresentation cases and pelvic ligament models to help make reasonable inferences about what examinees or diplomates do know about patient safety. For example, both the qualifying (written) and certifying (oral) examinations incorporate items and tasks assessing patient safety in order to help observe physicians' cognition of the topic. In addition, assessments and activities eliciting patient safety within the MOC program additionally assist with this component. Interpretations about diplomates' cognition and understanding on patient safety can then be extrapolated based on these observations. An extrapolation of this interpretation is the idea of implementation of patient safety (ie, candidates who have successfully mastered patient safety objectives can successfully practice safe medicine). **Fig. 2** shows this inter-relationship between cognition, observation, and interpretation, where diplomates' cognition of patient safety can be translated to their interpretation of it based on the observations made on ABOG's initial and continuous certification assessments.[7]

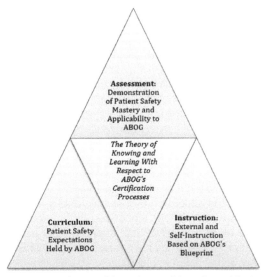

Fig. 1. Integrating Pellegrino's theory of knowing and learning with the ABOG's initial and continuing certification processes. (*Modified from* Pellegrino JW. The design of an assessment system for the race to the top: a learning sciences perspective on issues of growth and measurement. Explor Semin Meas Challenges Within Race to Top Agenda. Princeton, NJ, 2009: p. 1–37; with permission.)

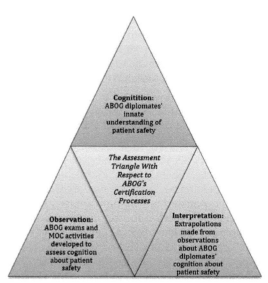

Fig. 2. Integrating Pellegrino's assessment triangle with ABOG's initial and continuing certification processes. (*Modified from* The nature of assessment and reasoning from evidence. In: Pellegrino JW, Chudowsky N, Glaser R, editors. Knowing what students know: the science and design of educational assessment. Washington, DC: National Academy Press; 2001; with permission.)

In the next sections, the authors describe ABOG's initial and continuous certification programs, and how principles of patient safety are intentionally embedded within its assessments and activities to evaluate the diplomates' understanding on patient safety.

INITIAL CERTIFICATION

Initial certification in obstetrics and gynecology by ABOG is a two-part process consisting of a computer-based qualifying examination and an oral certifying examination. This process improves women's health care by ensuring that candidates are striving for excellence in patient care across the spectrum of obstetrics and gynecology, by connecting cognition to interpretation by observation and assessment, as discussed in **Fig. 2**.

The Qualifying Examination

The qualifying examination can be taken at the completion of residency training. Candidates take a knowledge-based multiple choice computer examination that consists of 180 questions across the spectrum of obstetrics and gynecology. Patient safety and team-based care are intentionally embedded in the examination blueprint. Of the 180 questions, up to 10% explicitly and implicitly address patient safety. This amount has been relatively stable since the release of the ACGME core competencies in 1999. ABOG strives to test judgment, skills, and abilities in a more comprehensive fashion.

Starting in 2020, all candidates must have successfully completed the Fundamentals of Laparoscopic Surgery (FLS) course prior to taking the qualifying examination. The requirement of the FLS course for candidates is part of a larger initiative by the ABOG to incorporate simulation and standardize the knowledge and training completed by obstetric and gynecology residents. FLS is a validated, reliable, and comprehensive web-based education module offered by the Society of American Gastrointestinal and Endoscopic Surgeons (SAGES) that includes a hands-on skills training component and assessment tool designed to teach the physiology, fundamental knowledge, and technical skills required in basic laparoscopic surgery.[10,11] The incorporation of FLS into the initial certification process expands ABOG's ability to ensure candidates have achieved fundamental laparoscopic skills that will improve patient care.

The Certifying Examination

ABOG's certifying examination is taken after candidates have been in practice caring for their own patients for at least a year after completing residency training. In addition to structured cases that test across the spectrum of patient care, candidates are queried on the patients for whom they have cared.

To accurately assess the candidate's abilities in patient safety, specific structured cases are developed that test the candidate's judgment and skills. Candidates are required to explain how they incorporate all aspects of patient safety into their care of patients. For example, candidates may be asked to discuss immediate management and obligations of reporting for a case for which their colleague may not have surgical privileges. Another example would be a case dealing with a physician suffering from burnout and not providing appropriate care. The candidate may be asked to explain how he or she would engage the colleague and take over care to ensure that safe care was provided. The authors' hypothesis is that a candidate who is able to pass ABOG's certifying examination would receive fewer licensing actions, similar to the results from the study conducted by the American Board of Anesthesia.[12]

MAINTENANCE OF CERTIFICATION

The ABOG MOC program is a continuing professional development process to ensure that ABOG-certified physicians maintain a high level of knowledge, judgment, and skills in obstetrics, gynecology, and women's health throughout their careers. The program is a 6-year cycle that improves patient care by instituting high standards for continuous learning, practice improvement, and assessment activities of diplomates after achieving initial certification. During the 6-year cycle, diplomates will annually complete several requirements. After completion of a 6-year cycle, the process restarts the next year. There are 4 parts to the MOC process, but not all parts are active each year. The parts to the MOC program include:

- Part I: professionalism and professional standing
- Part II: lifelong learning and self-assessment
- Part III: assessment of knowledge, judgment, and skills
- Part IV: improvement in medical practice

The Standards for the ABMS Program for MOC were updated in 2014 and became effective in 2015.[13] The ABOG updated its MOC program in 2015 to meet these standards. The ABMS updates emphasized:

- Professionalism - how physicians carry out their responsibilities safely and ethically
- Patient safety - how physicians use patient safety knowledge to reduce harm and complications
- Performance improvement - how physicians use the best evidence and practices compared with peers and national benchmarks to treat patients

- Incorporating judgment into examinations - assessing not just what the physicians know but how they apply that knowledge

The components of MOC and how they address the ABMS standards are described next.

Maintenance of Certification Part I: Professionalism and Professional Standing

Board certification by the ABOG denotes that diplomates have demonstrated a commitment to patients' best interests, professional behavior, and adherence to certification requirements. A physician's professionalism and professional standing contribute to improved medical practice and help assure the public of better patient care. This includes:

1. Acting in patients' best interests
2. Behaving professionally with patients, families, and colleagues across health professions
3. Taking appropriate care of themselves
4. Representing their board certification and MOC status in a professional manner

ABOG requires an active, unrestricted license to practice medicine in any and all states or territories (United States or Canada) in which a physician is licensed as a measure of professionalism and professional standing. Diplomates must also uphold the moral and ethical standards of the practice of medicine accepted by organized medicine.

ABOG will query each state licensing board through the Federation of State Medical Boards (FSMB) for lists of physicians who hold active licenses.[14] Physician licensing, investigations of misconduct, and disciplinary actions occur at the state medical board level and are utilized by the ABOG to make decisions about diplomate eligibility to participate in MOC and disciplinary actions on certification status, which may include probation or loss of board certification

Maintenance of Certification Part II: Lifelong Learning and Self-Assessment

The primary goal of the ABOG MOC Part II Lifelong Learning and Self-Assessment is to encourage diplomates to read relevant and valuable journal articles and guidelines concerning clinical management and to encourage ABOG diplomates to develop a lifetime practice of learning.[14] This component of ABOG's MOC program has been in place since 1998 and was initially designated as the Annual Board Certification (ABC) process.

A foundational patient safety and communication course was developed in partnership by the American College of Obstetricians and Gynecologists (ACOG) and the ABOG in 2010 in order to meet the ABMS standards on patient safety. This course was incorporated into the MOC Part II assignments. The topics in the patient safety and communication course were relevant to the specialty of obstetrics and gynecology and included the following 14 chapters:

- Patient Safety: An Imperative
- A Just Culture
- Communication and Patient Safety
- Enhancing Patient Safety through Teamwork
- Medication Safety
- Disclosure of Adverse Events
- Medical Errors: Emotional Impact on Health Care Providers
- Leadership in Advancing Patient Safety

- High-Reliability Organizations
- Medical Errors and Near Misses: Performing Root Cause Analysis and Failure Mode and Effects Analysis
- Communication and Safety: Tracking and Reminder Systems
- Communication and Safety: Health Literacy
- Patient Safety in the Surgical Environment for the Obstetrician and Gynecologist
- Cultural Awareness and Sensitivity for the Practicing Obstetrician/Gynecologist

The patient safety and communication course was subsequently replaced by ABOG in 2015 with a new course that includes the following 8 chapters:

- Patient Safety: An Imperative
- Just Culture
- Enhancing Patient Safety through Teamwork
- Disclosure of Adverse Events
- Patient Safety in the Surgical Environment
- Medication Safety
- Communication and Patient Safety
- Cultural Awareness and Sensitivity for the Obstetrician - Gynecologist

In 2018, the patient safety and communication course was transitioned to an assessment-guided learning that incorporated patient safety journal articles in a new patient safety category within ABOG's MOC Part II Lifelong Learning and Self-Assessment. In order to offer important safety information with the aim to enhance lifelong learning, ABOG specialist and subspecialist diplomates are required to read 2 patient safety articles and answer questions each year to satisfy the patient safety requirement. Thus, over a 6-year MOC cycle, diplomates will read a total of 12 articles from the current literature on patient safety and answer 48 questions.

Partnerships with health care organizations enable ABOG to provide timely articles and guidelines on emerging topics in the MOC process. For example, the ABOG partnered with the US Centers for Disease Control and Prevention (CDC) in 2016 to help address the Zika virus public health care crisis by incorporating current and relevant articles into the Part II component of MOC. The ABOG also partners with ACOG and the ACOG Council on Patient Safety in Women's Health Care to include patient safety topics in MOC Part IV modules. Moreover, the ABOG utilizes subject matter experts to incorporate relevant articles in MOC Part II and modules in MOC Part IV. In 2018, several topics were added to the emerging topics category including opioid use during pregnancy, opioid prescribing after cesarean deliveries, and guidelines on Essure.

Maintenance of Certification Part III: Assessment of Knowledge, Judgment, and Skills

Assessment of Knowledge, Judgment and Skills (MOC Part III) builds upon and links to the continuous learning and self-assessment requirements of MOC Part II.[14] These standards contribute to better patient care and safety by integrating an external objective assessment to solidify a necessary commitment to lifelong learning and to remain current in core content of obstetrics and gynecology and its subspecialties. The examination blueprint is centered around topics such as diagnosis, decision-making, postoperative care and complications, and other relevant topics that physicians might encounter across a patient's care continuum. The ABOG specifically incorporates questions on the MOC Part III examination pertaining to how diplomates provide team-based care in order to improve their diagnostic abilities in some patient safety scenarios.

Maintenance of Certification Part IV: Improvement in Medical Practice

The ABMS approved new MOC standards in 2014 that encouraged member boards to ensure diplomates possess adequate knowledge of quality improvement (QI) science and practice.[13] These standards allowed the ABOG to expand the options for diplomates to demonstrate their commitment to improved patient care. Incorporation of these standards into MOC contributes to better patient care via ongoing self-assessment and improvement in the quality of care provided by diplomates. Until 2015, the only way a diplomate could meet the annual Part IV requirement was to complete an online module on a clinically relevant topic. ABOG created 4 additional pathways for MOC Part IV, which included QI activities, simulation courses, QI-related publications, and participation in the ABMS Multi-Specialty Portfolio Program (MSPP).[14] The additional pathways allowed ABOG to grant Part IV credit for the practice assessment activities in which many diplomates already participate within their practices, departments, hospitals, health systems, or community settings.

Diplomates complete an MOC Part IV Improvement in Medical Practice (IMP) activity annually in MOC years 1 to 5. There are currently 5 pathways available to allow diplomates to select the most clinically relevant option. An overview of each pathway is listed below:

1. IMP modules
   a. Evidence-based review followed by patient-related questions
   b. 150 topics in 9 clinically relevant categories
2. QI activities
   a. Well-designed QI projects based on accepted improvement science and methodology
3. Simulation
   a. Advanced, hands-on, clinical education experiences
4. QI-related publications, presentations, and posters
   a. Based on the results of QI projects
5. ABMS multispecialty portfolio program
   a. Alternate QI pathway available to sponsoring organizations that routinely oversee quality activities involving multiple medical specialties
   b. Provides a streamlined approach to providing MOC Part IV credit to multiple specialty boards by completing a single application

Improvement in medical practice modules

Although the popularity of Part IV alternative activities, such as simulation and QI efforts, continues to increase, most diplomates meet the annual requirement by selecting an IMP module, as shown in **Fig. 3**. The IMP module provides diplomates with an evidence-based review of the selected clinical topic and requires patient chart or administrative policy review. The chart review portion of the module allows the diplomate to complete a self-assessment, comparing his or her practice patterns to the clinical guidelines presented in the selected module. The practice profile questions are patient-specific and reflect the key points presented in the module. Diplomates are also required to submit feedback on whether the module influenced them to change their clinical practice and whether the topic was clinically relevant, valuable, and accurate. There are 9 IMP categories, including one on patient safety,

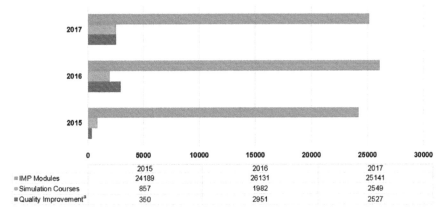

	2015	2016	2017
▪ IMP Modules	24189	26131	25141
▫ Simulation Courses	857	1982	2549
▪ Quality Improvement[a]	350	2951	2527

Fig. 3. Overview of MOC Part IV activity types selected by diplomates in 2015 to 2017. [a] Quality improvement is a combination of all approved QI pathways including ABOG-approved QI efforts, QI publications, presentations and posters, as well as the ABMS Portfolio Program.

communication, system-based practice, and ethics first offered in 2008. Currently the 12 modules in this category include:

- Abbreviations and symbols
- Cleaning and disinfection of intercavitary ultrasound transducers
- Disruptive behavior
- Fatigue and patient safety
- Informed consent
- Informed refusal
- Patient safety during surgery
- Relationships with the pharmaceutical and medical device industry
- Safe use of medications
- Sexual misconduct
- Tracking and reminder systems in the outpatient setting
- Ultrasound examination documentation

Quality improvement activities
QI activities are the result of identifying deficiencies in patient care and developing a plan of action to improve care through a series of interventions. ABOG-approved QI activities must address at least one of the Institute of Medicine (IOM) quality dimensions. The 6 quality dimensions state that health care should be safe, effective, patient-centered, timely, efficient, and equitable.[15] Since 2015, there are 5828 diplomates who have completed the MOC Part IV requirement by participating in one of the QI pathways. The expansion of Part IV alternatives in 2015 created an opportunity for ABOG to not only approve local QI efforts, but also national and state-level efforts. Perinatal quality collaboratives in several states have applied for QI credit for their members, and the ABOG also worked with ACOG to approve states that were participating in the Alliance for Innovation in Maternal Health (AIM) initiative. The ABOG also serves as a member of the ACOG Women's Health Registry Alliance and coordinated with several women's health registries to grant MOC Part IV credit to diplomates for meaningful participation in clinical outcomes registries.

   The CDC is coordinating with many states and jurisdictions to develop task forces to address maternal mortality issues. The CDC requested that ABOG recognize the committee members for their efforts to improve women's health care. In 2018, the ABOG implemented the granting of MOC Part IV credit to diplomates who are members of maternal mortality and morbidity review committees.

Simulation

The ABOG created the simulation pathway for MOC Part IV to promote simulation as a valuable training tool linked to improved clinical outcomes through the continuum of training and clinical practice.[16,17] Hands-on simulation courses are increasingly offered at national meetings and on a local-level for team and unit training. The ABOG partners with specialty societies to approve these courses each year. Multidisciplinary team training in a simulated environment improves communication and teamwork skills during critical events. Participants benefit from simulating life-threatening events in a learner-friendly environment. Simulation training is associated with improved clinical outcomes in several obstetric emergencies such as shoulder dystocia, postpartum hemorrhage, and emergent cesarean delivery.[16] More than 5300 diplomates have received simulation credit for MOC Part IV since 2015.

Quality improvement publications, presentations, and posters

ABOG awards MOC Part IV credit to diplomates for peer-reviewed publications, oral presentations, and posters presented at national scientific meetings that outline the process and results of quality improvement initiatives in health care. The QI project should address a recognized gap in care, generally be prospective, and involve more than 1 QI cycle. This pathway for MOC Part IV was created because ABOG recognized the importance of physicians sharing their experience implementing QI initiatives. Diplomates can potentially gain insight to solving a similar health care issue and could replicate successful interventions within their own practice.

American Board of Medical Specialties Portfolio Program

The ABMS Multi-Specialty Portfolio Program is an alternative pathway for health care organizations that support physician involvement in QI. Most portfolio program QI activities are sponsored by the institution or hospital QI departments. They are typically multispecialty, system-wide initiatives, although they may be obstetrics and gynecology specific. This pathway offers a streamlined approach to MOC Part IV for hospitals and health systems that may complete an application for multiple specialties.

SUMMARY

The ABOG is a nonprofit organization that certifies obstetricians and gynecologists and also offers continuous certification (MOC) to obstetricians and gynecologists in the United States and Canada. The mission of the ABOG is to define specialty standards, certify obstetricians and gynecologists, and facilitate continuous learning to advance knowledge, practice, and professionalism in women's health. Patient safety content is embedded into the assessments within the initial certification process and within the continuous certification process by ABOG to ensure as much as possible that diplomates practice safely. Patient safety journal articles and modules were intentionally incorporated in the content of continuous certification in 2018 at the ABOG to offer important safety information throughout lifelong learning for diplomates. In addition, observational tools are developed within initial and continuous certification (such as assessments and simulations) so that diplomates' cognition of patient safety can be extrapolated to implementation. For example, improvement in medical practice was integrated into the ABOG's Maintenance of Certification Program. Improving medical practice influences better quality patient care via continuing assessment and advancement in the quality of care in physicians' office practices, hospitals, and health systems.

Given the ever-evolving field of health care, the ABOG remains committed to continually assessing and adapting its initial and continuing certification programs to include patient safety concepts and ensure that women are receiving quality health care from ABOG diplomates.

REFERENCES

1. American Board of Medical Specialties. ABMS Home. About us. Available at: https://www.abms.org. Accessed September 18, 2018.
2. American Board of Medical Specialties. ABMS/NPSF issue joint call for patient safety activities. Press Release. Available at: https://www.abms.org/news-events/abmsnpsf-issue-joint-call-for-patient-safety-activities/. Accessed September 18, 2018.
3. American Board of Medical Specialties. Measuring competence in quality and safety. Patient safety. Available at: https://www.abms.org/news-events/measuring-competence-in-quality-and-safety/?cat=patient-safety. Accessed July 20, 2017.
4. Bransford JD, Brown AL, Cocking RR, et al. How people learn: brain, mind, experience, and school. In: Bransford JD, Brown AL, Cocking RR, et al, editors. Expanded edition. Washington, DC: National Academies Press; 2000. p. 51–78.
5. Donovan MS, Bransford JD. How students learn history, science and mathematics in the classroom. In: Donovan MS, Bransford JD, editors. Washington, DC: National Academies Press; 2005. p. 1–28.
6. Donovan MS, Bransford JD, Pellegrino JW. How people learn: bridging research and practice. In: Donovan MS, Bransford JD, Pellegrino JW, editors. Washington, DC: National Academies Press; 1999. p. 10–24.
7. Pellegrino JW, Chudowsky N, Glaser R. Knowing what students know: the science and design of educational assessment. In: Pellegrino JW, Chudowsky N, Glaser R, editors. Washington, DC: National Academies Press; 2001. p. 37–56.
8. Shepard LA. The role of assessment in a learning culture. Educ Res 2000;29(7): 4–14.
9. Pellegrino JW. The design of an assessment system for the race to the top: a learning sciences perspective on issues of growth and measurement. Explor Semin Meas Challenges Within Race to Top Agenda. Princeton, NJ, 2009 (December 2009): p. 1–37. https://doi.org/10.1002/tea.20324.
10. Vassiliou MC, Dunkin BJ, Marks JM, et al. FLS and FES: comprehensive models of training and assessment. Surg Clin North Am 2010;90(3):535–58.
11. Society of American Gastrointestinal and Endoscopic Surgeons. Fundamentals of laparoscopic surgery. Available at: www.flsprogram.org. Accessed October 31, 2018.
12. Zhou Y, Sun H, Culley DJ, et al. Effectiveness of written and oral specialty certification examinations to predict actions against the medical licenses of anesthesiologists. Anesthesiology 2017;126(6):1171–9.
13. American Board of Medical Specialties. Standards for the ABMS Program for Maintenance of Certification (MOC). Available at: https://www.abms.org/media/1109/standards-for-the-abms-program-for-moc-final.pdf Accessed October 24, 2018.
14. American Board of Obstetrics and Gynecology. ABOG specialty maintenance of certification bulletin. Available at: https://www.abog.org/docs/default-source/

abog-bulletins/2018-moc-specialty-bulletin.pdf?sfvrsn=91d29c24_2. Accessed October 24, 2018.

15. Institute of Medicine (US). Committee on Quality of Health Care in America. Crossing the quality chasm : a new health system for the 21st century. Washington, DC: National Academy Press; 2001.

16. Satin AJ. Medical education: clinical expert series simulation in obstetrics. Obstet Gynecol 2018;132:199–209.

17. Gavin NR, Satin AJ. Simulation training in obstetrics. Clin Obstet Gynecol 2017; 60(4):802–10.

Implementing Patient Safety Initiatives

Paul James Armand Ruiter, BMSc, MD, MCFP

KEYWORDS

- Patient safety • Implementation • Engagement • Safety II • Resilience
- Interprofessional • Ownership

KEY POINTS

- Engagement in health care is a challenge.
- Current concepts of patient safety have changed.
- Implementation of initiatives requires an understanding of the current context, in both engagement and safety. An approach based on experience from the MORE[OB] Program, with more than 300 birthing teams will be presented.

INTRODUCTION

Implementing change is challenging. However, successful implementation is possible and once achieved, is rewarding.

Success requires a clear understanding of:

- Health care context
- Patient safety
- Behavioral psychology

To achieve its goal, this article is divided into 3 parts:

- *The Problem with Engagement in Healthcare*: the issues affecting engagement of health care workers.
- *Patient Safety in a New Age*: patient safety in the context of complexity science and human behavior.
- *Implementation:* a simple, deliberate, and reproducible process that respects context and complexity.

Disclosure: Dr P.J.A. Ruiter is the Medical Director and Vice President of the Salus Global Corporation, a company in business to research and develop Patient Safety and Quality Improvement Programs.

Salus Global, Knowledge Translation & Implementation Science Faculty, Canadian Patient Safety Institute, 200 - 717 Richmond Street, London, Ontario N6A 1S2, Canada

E-mail address: James.Ruiter@SalusGlobal.com

IMPLEMENTING PATIENT SAFETY INITIATIVES

Successful implementation of change requires active and willing participation called *engagement*.

PART 1: THE PROBLEM WITH ENGAGEMENT IN HEALTH CARE

In 2015, only 57% of health care workers considered themselves *engaged:* 10% less than 5 years before. Thirty percent of the health care workers considered themselves as *just contributing* and 13% called themselves either *actively disengaged* or *hostile*.[1] These figures have been steadily worsening over years.

In 2018, 50 senior leaders, middle managers, educators, and front-line workers in a 55-hospital health system came together to discuss improving quality of care and life at work. The TRIZ method, a process in which participants list components of initiatives that undermine engagement, provided insight.[2] Every item, from the extensive list assembled that could contribute to disengagement, was present within their initiatives.

Inadvertently, the system has evolved to disengage its employees.

Contributing Factors

The program of the week
Everyone desires a quick fix. These have led to a revolving door of programs, known to staff as *"the flavor of the week."* Reinforced by regulating bodies' requirements, this is also known as *Institutional Attention Deficit Disorder* (Gardam M, personal communication, 2018). It is further accentuated by the high turnover of senior leadership. In health care, CEO turnover ranged from 16% to 20% between 2011 and 2015.[1] New CEOs want things done their way, which leads to changes in processes and programs leaving insufficient time for anything to have an impact.

Just get it done The perceived easiest way to implement change is a mandate to the staff. This approach seldom works. Much of what is needed to improve health care is already described; it just needs to be implemented! Mandates do not lead to sustainable solutions or a strong team and likely contribute to disengagement.[3,4]

Buy-in—is it truly what is wanted? Leaders often seek *buy-in* from their health care teams. This is not what leaders actually want.

When we seek *buy-in,* we are asking colleagues to accept an idea that was developed with minimal input from the team it affects.[5] Leaders rationalize that their colleagues were too busy to provide input. In fact, leaders did not give them the opportunity to contribute. Thus, leaders seek the team's acceptance of an externally created process.

Successful *buy-in* means that the team is content to follow orders. It is a sign of an unhealthy organization and of a disengaged workforce with decreased mindfulness.[5] If something goes wrong, the team will attribute the problem to the leader and reject accountability. The team becomes part of the problem. Such change, imposed by others, is often overtly or covertly opposed.[6]

Safety and quality
Describing Safety as distinct from Quality is as describing *Bananas* as distinct from *Fruit.* It has severed Safety from Quality.[7] As a result, many of us have witnessed excellent, evidence-based processes that may not be safe in certain contexts:

- In the physical design of our unit,
- In combination with existing processes,

- In the target population, and
- In our locale.

Safety must be integral to quality. If not, front-line providers will not engage.

Data swamp and its impact

We are in a data glut. "In pursuit of incentives, we've glutted ourselves with metrics. I think we are way beyond a level of toxicity. It's not just safety. We have to go on a diet."[7]

Furthermore, Benchmarks and Key Performance Indicators have had unintended consequences and have led to "perverse outcomes."[6,8]

Finally, teams often have data used against them. They are penalized for a high cesarean section rate and loose funding for low unit census.

We need to flip data on its head.

Data must drive engagement and become a reward. What is measured must be relevant, timely, and usable by the team making the change (*Leading Indicators*).[9]

PART 2: PATIENT SAFETY IN A NEW AGE

The year 2019 marks the twentieth anniversary of the presentation to Congress of the Institute of Medicine's report: *To Err is Human*.[10] Although not the first, it was the most widely publicized report on preventable harm in health care. Subsequent studies came to similar conclusions.[11,12]

Despite pockets of excellence, the numbers of harm keep rising.[13,14] Although we have been arguing over the numbers, "action and progress on patient safety is frustratingly slow."[13] The overall harm rate remains 10%.[6]

Why?

Humans are inattentive

Classified as cognition errors, these tend to be memory slips and lapses. For example: *I misdial my mother's phone number.* The frequent response to these errors is "retraining." This does little to reduce the likelihood of recurrence.

Humans make mistakes

Retraining may help here. Both "inattentiveness" and "mistakes" benefit from a *Just Culture*, which postulates for cognition-based errors, the health care worker should be consoled unless there is deliberate and wilful violation of safety guidelines. In that case, irrespective of patient harm, sanctions and punishment are necessary (David Marx's article, "Patient Safety and the Just Culture," in this issue).

Humans routinely bend or break rules

"Social normalization of deviance" means that people within the organization become accustomed to bending the rules and consider it normal.[15]

Should this behavior be punished when some deviations may improve safety by finding new ways to improve complex processes?

What factors encouraged the health care team to behave in that way? Can every rule be followed? Is every deviance bad?

Deviance

Deviance is ubiquitous in all human endeavors. Work has 4 dimensions:

- Work as Imagined—as a nonclinical CEO might imagine the process of delivering a baby.

- Work as Prescribed—where a work process is created: policies, procedures, or guidelines.
- Work as Done—how the work prescribed is actually performed by those who do the work.
- Work as Disclosed—how the work is reported to have been done.[16]

In health care, these 4 dimensions are rarely concordant.[17]

What causes this difference? Work is often prescribed for frontline workers by review of best practices and by individuals not directly involved. This leads to disconnect from reality. The process needs to be adapted and made to work within the local environment, by those who do the work: the front line.[17] Furthermore, there are far too many rules for anyone to remember, look up, keep up-to-date, or follow.[18,19] At best, in only 40% of cases are all the rules followed despite the use of bundles and checklists.[20]

Hospitals are stressed by production pressure (economic, workload...).[21] This need to continually "produce" leads the organization to seek *efficiency* at the expense of *thoroughness*.[22] In this light, it is not possible for Work as Done to resemble Work as Imagined or Work as Prescribed.[17]

In this way, the organization gives tacit approval to Work as Done, until something goes wrong. When, in hindsight, it realizes the team should have been more thorough in that one instance.[22] The worker is often held accountable to an unachievable rule within the existing context. Often, the erroneous conclusion is that the deviation caused the harm. But in a complex multidimensional care environment the results might have been the same even if the rule was followed. As a final consequence of this approach, 2 things are likely to follow: another new policy to prevent recurrence is created and the original rule remains unaltered. Staff remains disengaged; harm is not reduced.

Care is not linear

Policies incorrectly infer that care is *linear* and workload *average*. Despite advances in complexity theory, models that infer linearity, such as the "Swiss Cheese" model of harm causality, persist.[23]

Care is multidimensional and tightly coupled.[21] Hence, linear theories, which produce linear protective safety rules (policies, procedures) will often not work because the sequences of events may never recur in that same way again. These solutions can have unintended consequences: the diversion of resources from other tasks, increased risk in other areas, and inefficiency (Kotaska A, personal communication, 2018).

What Is Safety?

Safety has traditionally been seen as a nonevent: if nothing bad has happened, the patient was safe. Measuring this nonevent is impossible.[24] This is supported by current Safety Management, which "is based on analyzing situations where something went wrong."[25] Safety Management expects stability, certainty, and predictability and seeks to control, manage, and restrict to *engineer-out* failure (know as Protective Safety or Safety I).[26] Yet modern day health care does not function in stable, certain, and predictable environments. Nor does it function on stable, certain, and predictable patients with stable conditions. The status quo safety solution—treating health care as an aircraft carrier or a nuclear power plant—is incongruent to the real environment it purports to protect. It is therefore highly likely that the sole approach of *engineering-out* failure, with more safety rules, in a Complex and Adaptive System is not an effective or engaging method to increase safety.[27]

Complex challenges require a different approach, one that combines critical examination of the system's components balanced with an understanding of the interaction of its workers.[28] We must create resilient organizations that "absorb" and catch errors and limit the damage when they do occur, instead of just being reactionary (Gardam M, personal communication, 2018), and[29] this requires combining the traditional focus of Protective Safety with that of Productive Safety or *engineering-in success* (which views Safety as the dynamic event of a case gone well), understanding why care went well, and increasing the likelihood of future successes.[17,24,30,31]

Culture

Organizational culture has been identified as the critical factor to accelerate improvements in patient safety.[32] Because achieving the right culture is difficult, the usual choice of health care is to accept and work within the existing default culture.

Culture is often described as *"what we do around here,"* but it is also *"what we choose to tolerate."* In that light, each one of us has a critical role in promoting a safe culture. Quality improvement within health care should focus on achieving that culture. A positive correlation has been shown between culture and patient outcomes.[33–35]

Safety tools

Knowledge moves in 3 sequential phases: Superficial Simplicity, Confusing Complexity, and Profound Simplicity.[32] Safety in health care is currently at the stage of Confusing Complexity:

Superficial Simplicity: early work in safety believed that adapting some of the tools from the airline industry—a complicated system—would lead to great improvements in health care quality and safety.

Confusing Complexity: the current state of safety in health care: more than 600 + policies, guidelines, and procedures guide workers in 1 day at the average hospital.[18]

Profound Simplicity: the right balance of guides, operationally informed by an understanding of the system and its people.

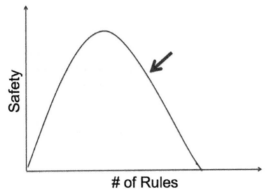

Fig. 1. Beyond an optimal number of safety rules in the environment, safety begins to erode.

"Too many safety rules can overwhelm, and frustrate a worker, enabling danger to emerge."[26] There are an optimal number of safety rules. Safety degrades if there are too few or too many. Currently, as arbitrarily indicated by the arrow, we are beyond the ideal number (**Fig. 1**) (Gluck P, personal communication, 2017).

Complexity of the System and Its Patients

Health care is a Complex Adaptive System in contrast with Simple and Complicated Systems. This is best explained as follows:[9]

A *Simple System* is baking a cake:

- Following a list of linear tasks results in a cake.
- Features: the process can be easily taken apart, understood, rebuilt, and the desired outcome repeatedly achieved.
- Safety systems to prevent failure include ingredient lists, standardized tools, and a process (recipe).

A *Complicated System* is placing a human on the moon:

- Highly involved linear and multilinear tasks must be completed in the correct order and followed to the minute detail.
- Features: the process can be broken down, understood, rebuilt, and the desired outcome repeatedly achieved.
- Safety systems to prevent failure include checklists, standardization, and rigorous attention to detail.

A *Complex System* is raising a child:

- Features: the process cannot be broken down, understood, and rebuilt to achieve the same outcome. Raising each child is different.
- In raising a child, parents work to *engineer-in* success by applying general principles or simple rules that increase the likelihood of a good outcome.

Although safety rules for complicated systems work in simple systems, neither system's safety rules work in complex systems. They may actually cause harm through unintended consequences.[30] Furthermore, solutions in Complex Adaptive Systems cannot be applied unchanged to the next department. Context, complexity, and local culture must be considered.[36] This explains why some attempts at standardization fail.

Finally, Complex Adaptive Systems meet the needs of their unpredictably changing contexts through workers' flexibility and ingenuity, often restricted by current safety approaches.[27]

Although health care is a Complex Adaptive System, it also contains elements of Simple and Complicated systems. Improvements in safety require a balancing of the right safety tool for the right part of the system.

PART 3: IMPLEMENTATION—PUTTING IT ALL TOGETHER

To affect meaningful and sustainable change, it is essential to reengage front-line staff. To do so, they need to know that their input is valued and results in timely and relevant change.[28,34,37] The front-line team must help identify the problem, own the problem, and together find and implement effective solutions.[34] Leadership must support this approach by building infrastructure and capacity.[38]

The Rebuilding of Engagement

Front-line *Ownership* requires an understanding of how the work is actually done and the impact of changes.[5,27,28,38] This approach needs leadership guidance, nurture, support, and time. Once established, the unit will be transformed from reactive to proactive.[35,39]

What is required is a small representative interprofessional core group from the hospital unit.[40,41] Ideally it is a self-organized heterarchy and represents every professional group working on the unit.[27] Its role is to select and prioritize relevant improvement projects, develop the intervention, and manage its roll out.[35] The core group must be nurtured and empowered by leadership:

Nurture: only the organization can provide the *capacity* for the team to exercise its newfound *capability.*

Empower: early *quick-wins* built into the plan will rally the rest of the department and encourage the core group to continue its work. Turnover of the core group is important for new ideas, to prevent burnout, sustain change, and prevent them from being seen as a new hierarchy.

Leadership: leadership of the core group should be by front-line staff—having co-chairs is optimal. The group should include department leaders to facilitate and accelerate identified change.

The Reintegration of Safety into Quality

The project chosen must be relevant to the unit as a whole and not seen as *top-down*. This helps develop ownership.[28] A Continuous Quality Improvement (CQI) approach sustains knowledge and helps reunite safety with quality.[41] Every project purposefully advances the unit's goal.

The core group should initially focus on known safety gaps to ensure relevance, allow for quick-wins, and develop comfort in the core group's growing abilities. As the group matures, previously unidentified but relevant gaps, discovered through worker surveys, debrief recommendations, and analyzing No-Harm events, should be addressed. This proactive approach builds a positive culture and reengages staff.[35]

Key elements of the CQI framework (**Fig. 2**) are:

- Education: what is the gap the team wants to address?
- Evaluation: is the gap relevant to the unit/department? What measures would reflect success? A few relevant measures that will indicate early successes, known as leading indicators or pulse point, are important.[36] They are a reward for engagement, are prioritized over other measures, and their achievement should be celebrated.[3]
- Practice Modification/Process Improvement: this is the intervention, led by the core group to close the gap. It requires individual learning, coupled with application of this knowledge (through "processing" by every profession) to the specific environment of that unit.[5,39,42] Tools to facilitate this knowledge transfer include interprofessional unit-wide workshops, case discussions, or in-situ simulations,[35,39,43] all designed to challenge the status quo and reconcile Work as Prescribed with Work as Done.[39,41]
- Reflection occurs as the outcomes and the processes of change are evaluated. An understanding of what worked well, and what did not, makes the core group more effective as it approaches each new project.

At least 1 or 2 recommendations with measurable impact that are easy to implement should be initiated quickly. An important quick-win, this visible action by leadership

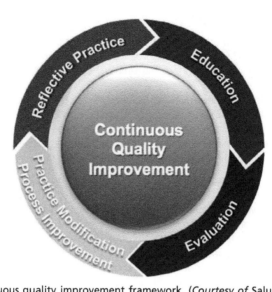

Fig. 2. A continuous quality improvement framework. (*Courtesy of* Salus Global, Ontario, Canada.)

helps reverse the trend toward disengagement and is critical for the success of the core group.[37,44] Conversely, if the core group's initial actions fail, frontline workers will become even less engaged.[27,44]

As part of an intervention, in-situ simulations should challenge linear thinking. They offer an opportunity to stress organizational processes and safety boundaries.[45] If done with attention to psychological safety, individual perspectives are revealed that foster awareness of the interdependencies among professionals, essential for successful quality improvement and organizational resilience.[28,45] Furthermore, simulations can build trust and improve interprofessional team culture.[35,43]

All interventions must reconcile Work as Done with Work as Prescribed. Comments such as "It is all well and good that our policy says X, but we had Mrs Smith here last week, and we did Y" are key moments that set the stage for meaningful improvement.[5]

The purpose for the core group's activities must be clearly communicated. All stakeholders are informed how each individual activity relates to the improvement goals.[44]

The core group needs a coach. This partnership is accountable for implementation of the safety improvement plan. The coach should have expertise in the area of improvements in complex adaptive systems. The core group understands how best to apply these strategies to the unit context and culture.[27]

Coaches may be external consultants or hospital employees. Objective, external consultants may be better positioned to address barriers for successful implementation.

Measuring engagement of the wider unit team, in the intervention designed and executed by the core group, is in itself an important leading indicator of movement toward a culture of patient safety.

OTHER CONSIDERATIONS THAT CAN HELP BUILD ENGAGEMENT
Routine Debriefing of Normal Cases

Debriefs are valuable in learning not only from cases where care should be improved but also from cases where care went well.

Debriefing of events, irrespective of patient harm, allows the team to learn from mistakes and improve processes. A simple example: a forceps-assisted operative vaginal delivery is required. Two left blades are provided in the set, preventing you from completing the procedure. Quickly, your team obtains a second set; this time a left and a right blade allow you to complete the delivery. A traditional approach, if the event is even reported, identifies the Latent Factors[23] that facilitated the event to occur. Processes are put in place to prevent the already unlikely recurrence of 2 same blades in a set. This is Protection Safety or Safety I.

Debriefing of successes helps the team develop the skill to replicate the care for other scenarios, shedding more light on Work as Done. In this way, debriefing the case of the 2 left blades would identify not only the Latent Factors but also the features of the team that prevented harm. These features are leveraged and built upon, allowing the team to be resilient and proactive when faced with other challenges. This approach reduces the stigma of only discussing the "bad."

Improving process solely as a result of negative events will make quality improvement an episodic occurrence with a negative context.

Debriefing when cases go well builds a positive culture while allowing for potential improvements in an already good process.[17] Quality improvement must be continuous not episodic. This approach forms the basis of Productive Safety or Safety II: Improving Quality by increasing successful outcomes, improving culture, and the work environment.[35,44,46]

Understanding why we succeed is as important as understanding why we fail. Balancing these 2 sides of the safety equation—a balance that is unique for every unit—allows the leveraging of the strengths of our workforce as well as improving its weaknesses.

Therefore, classic risk management focuses on episodic failures and tends to regard people as the problem. Newer thinking (Safety II, Productive Safety) seeks to also understand Work as Done and learn from successes. It regards people as the resource that adapts to unexpected situations, and tries to understand how those learnings can be incorporated into fewer, yet better and more nimble processes.[17,22]

Improving safety by increasing the likelihood of things going right rather than focusing on the few cases of harm is not a competing viewpoint. Increasing the likelihood of things going right reduces the harm rate.[18] These are simply 2 opposite ends of the same performance teeter-totter (**Fig. 3**). Focusing on increasing what is done right is more

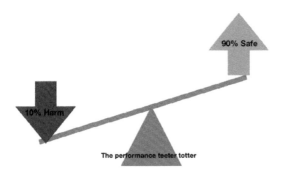

Fig. 3. The performance teeter-totter: increasing the 90% of what goes right effectively decreases the occurrence of harm.

achievable, cost-effective,[34] and engages more people by creating a positive culture.[17] However, there is a balance between the 2 approaches, which is different in every unit.

SUMMARY

Safety is all about cultures that promote engagement and facilitates relevant change.[27,32,34,35] Recognizing that health care is a complex adaptive system, the process described will lead units to that culture by design.[35] Complex systems evolve over years in response to their unique environment. Their successful performance is inextricably linked to their culture.

Although parts of the health care system are simple and some are complicated, the largest components are complex and adaptive. Future advances in safety and quality require us to strike a balance between regarding the human element as a liability and as a resource.

Positive, relevant, and timely change will rebuild the engagement of our workforce to bring about renewed successes in Patient Safety. We need to work with our complex system, not against it. Every one of us holds an important role in achieving that goal.

REFERENCES

1. Quantum, employee engagement in healthcare industry report. Available at: https://www.quantumworkplace.com/employee-engagement-in-healthcare. Accessed March 20, 2018.
2. Liberating structures. Available at: http://www.liberatingstructures.com/6-making-space-with-triz/. Accessed April 12, 2017.
3. Gardam M, Gitterman L, Rykert L, et al. Healthcare quality improvement requires many approaches. Healthc Pap 2017;17(1):57–61.
4. Flanagan ME, Welsh CA, Kiss C, et al. A national collaborative for reducing health care associated infections: current initiatives, challenges and opportunities. Am J Infect Control 2011;38(8):685–9.
5. Zimmerman B, Reason P, Rykert L, et al. Front-line ownership: generating a cure mindset for patient safety. Healthc Pap 2013;13(1):6–22.
6. Braithwaitte J. Changing how we think about healthcare improvement. BMJ 2018; 361:k2014.
7. Berwick D, O'Connor M. Don Berwick's 7 roadblocks to improving patient safety 2017. Available at: https://www.hhnmag.com/articles/8310-don-berwicks-7-roadblocks-to-improving-patient-safety. Accessed May 20, 2017.
8. Mannion R, Braithwaite J. Unintended consequences of performance measurement in healthcare: 20 salutary lessons from the English National Health Service. Intern Med J 2012;42:569–74.
9. Gardam M. The complex road to lasting change. In Breakfast for the Chiefs proceedings. 2017. Available at: http://www.longwoods.com/audio-video/all/1/7607. Accessed October 18, 2017.
10. Kohn LT, Corrigan JM, Donaldson MS, editors. To err is human: building a safer health system. Washington, DC: National Academy Press; 2000. p. 1663. Available at: https://www.nationalacademies.org/hmd/~/media/Files/Report%20Files/1999/To-Err-is-Human/To%20Err%20is%20Human%201999%20%20report%20brief.pdf. Accessed October 15, 2016.
11. Baker GR, Norton P, Flintoft V, et al. The Canadian adverse events study: the incidence of adverse events among hospital patients in Canada. CMAJ 2004; 170(11):1678–86.

12. Department of Health. An organisation with a memory: report of an expert group on learning from adverse events in the NHS. London: The Stationary Office; 2000.
13. James JT. A new, evidence-based estimate of patient harms associated with hospital care. J Patient Saf 2013;9(3):122–8.
14. Makary MA, Daniel M. Medical error-the third leading cause of death in the US. BMJ 2016;353:i2139.
15. Vaughan D. Sociologist, Columbia University, Consultant May 2008. Available at: http://www.consultingnewsline.com/Info/Vie%20du%20Conseil/Le%20Consultant%20du%20mois/Diane%20Vaughan%20(English).html. Accessed August 28, 2018.
16. Ombredane A, Faverge JM. L'analyse du travail. Paris: Presses Universitaires de France; 1955.
17. Hollnagel E. In safety-I and safety-II. London: Ashgate; 2014.
18. Braithwaite J. Resilient health care: reconciling work-as-imagined and work-as-done. Proceedings from leading together: achieving results, Canadian conference on physician leadership 2016. Available at: http://physicianleaders.ca. Accessed June 10, 2016.
19. Amalberti R. Patient safety as a moving target: implications for improvement strategies. Proceedings from the 1st Latin-American Forum - ISQua. Cartagena de Indias, Colombia, May 18, 2016.
20. Redesigning Care—A new playbook to improve quality, safety and patient-centered care, Proceedings from the 23rd annual health and forum and the American hospital association leadership summit. San Francisco, July 25, 2016.
21. Cook R, Rasmussen J. "Going solid:" a model of system dynamics and consequences for patient safety. Qual Saf Health Care 2005;14:130–4.
22. Hollnagel E. The ETTO principle: efficiency-thoroughness trade-off. London: Taylor and Francis Group; 2009.
23. Reason J. Managing the risk of organisational accidents. Aldershot (UK): Ashgate Publishing; 1997.
24. Stænder S. Safety-II and resilience: the way ahead in patient safety in anaesthesiology. Curr Opin Anaesthesiol 2015;28. https://doi.org/10.1097/ACO.0000000000000252.
25. Hollnagel E. Resilience in healthcare from proceedings from annual CCSO quality conference Toronto. Ontario, Canada, March 23, 2016.
26. Wong G. 7 Implications of complexity for safety. 2018. Available at: http://www.safetydifferently.com/7-implications-of-complexity-for-safety/. Accessed April 5, 2018.
27. Braithwaite J, Churruca K, Ellis LA, et al. Complexity science in healthcare – aspirations, approaches, applications and accomplishments: a white paper. Sydney (Australia): Australian Institute of Health Innovation, Macquarie University; 2017.
28. Gardam M, Gitterman L, Rykert L, et al. Five years of experience using front-line ownership to improve healthcare quality and safety. Healthc Pap 2017;17(1):7–23.
29. Knox EG, Rice Simpson K. Perinatal high reliability. Am J Obstet Gynecol 2011;204(5):373–7.
30. Johnson A. Framework for better care; Proceedings from the 6th resilient health care meeting. University of British Columbia, British Columbia, Canada, August 15, 2017.
31. Decker S. Why do things go right? Safety differently. Available at: http://www.safetydifferently.com/why-do-things-go-right/. Accessed September 29, 2018.

32. Free from harm, accelerating patient safety improvement fifteen years after to Err is human, expert panel report. The National Patient Safety Foundation; 2015. Available at: http://www.ihi.org/resources/Pages/Publications/Free-from-Harm-Accelerating-Patient-Safety-Improvement.aspx. Accessed January 2016.

33. Braithwaite J, Herkes J, Ludlow K, et al. Association between organisational and workplace cultures, and patient outcomes: systematic review. BMJ Open 2017;7: e017708.

34. Geary M, Ruiter PJA, Yasseen AS III. Examining the effects of an obstetrics inter-professional programme on reductions to reportable events and their related costs. J Interprof Care 2018. https://doi.org/10.1080/13561820.2018.1543255.

35. Accreditation Canada, the Healthcare Insurance Reciprocal of Canada, the Ca-nadian Medical Protective Association, Salus Global Corporation. Obstetrics ser-vices in Canada: advancing quality and strengthening safety. Ottawa (Canada): Accreditation Canada; 2016.

36. Blignaut S. Seven implications of complexity for organisations, More Beyond. Available at: https://www.morebeyond.co.za/7-implications-of-complexity-for-organisations/. Accessed March 20, 2018.

37. Bailey S, Bevan H. Quality improvement: lessons from the English National Health Services. Healthc Pap 2017;17(1):49–55.

38. Carney B, Getz I. Give your team the freedom to do the work they think matters most. Harvard Business Review 2018. Available at: https://hbr.org/2018/09/give-your-team-the-freedom-to-do-the-work-they-think-matters-most.

39. Ruiter PJ, Cameron C. Birth models that nurture cooperation between profes-sionals: pizza and other keys to disarmament. In: Daviss BA, Davis-Floyd R, editors. Speaking truth to power: childbirth models on the human rights frontier. London: University of California Press; 2019. p. 9.

40. Lanham HJ, Leykum LK, Taylor BS, et al. How complexity science can inform scale-up and spread in health care: understanding the role of self-organization in variation across local contexts. Soc Sci Med 2013;93:194–202.

41. Burke C, Grobman W, Miller D. Interdisciplinary collaboration to maintain a culture of safety in a labor and delivery setting. J Perinat Neonatal Nurs 2013;27(2): 113–23.

42. Minshall T. University of Cambridge Research: what is knowledge transfer. Avail-able at: http://www.cam.ac.uk/research/news/what-is-knowledge-transfer. Ac-cessed May 15, 2017.

43. Macrae C, Draycott T. Delivering high reliability in maternity care: in situ simula-tion as a source of organisational resilience. Saf Sci 2016. https://doi.org/10.1016/j.ssci.2016.10.019.

44. Ruiter PJ. In-Situ simulation - a practical guide, reflections on low-tech simulation after 17 years of MOREOB, Forthcoming 2019.

45. Leykum L, Kumar P, Parchman M, et al. Use of an agent-based model to under-stand clinical systems. J Artif Soc Soc Simul 2012;15(3). https://doi.org/10.18564/jasss.1905.

46. Decker S. Safety differently. Available at: https://www.youtube.com/watch?v=moh4QN4IAPg. Accessed November 20, 2017.

Leadership and Teamwork
Essential Roles in Patient Safety

John P. Keats, MD, CPE, CPPS*

KEYWORDS

- Culture • Vision • Direction-setting • Standardization • Communication
- Situational awareness • Team learning

KEY POINTS

- Medical care has become increasingly complex and potentially unsafe.
- Leadership and teamwork are the foundations of patient safety.
- Leadership improves safety by creating a vision and setting organizational direction within a patient-centric culture.
- Teamwork improves safety by establishing norms of communication and situational awareness.

INTRODUCTION

Since its founding, medical care has undergone a fundamental transformation in this country. "Medicine used to be simple, ineffective, and relatively safe. It is now complex, effective, and potentially dangerous."[1] Modern environments for the provision of health care have become increasingly complex with computer-aided technologies, combined with patients with higher rates of chronic illness, obesity, and comorbidities. Obstetrics and gynecology are practiced in complex environments. Surgical procedures are fraught with the potential for patient harm including anesthesia complications, excessive blood loss, unintended injury to adjacent structures, and accidental retention of sponges or surgical instruments. Labor units, which combine elements of an emergency room, operating room, and intensive care unit, are especially problematic.

How can one maintain a safe environment for patients amid all this complexity? The foundation for safe health care is effective teamwork striving toward a common goal. "The mystical authority of the doctor used to be essential for practice. Now we need to be open and work in partnership with our colleagues in health care and with our patients."[1] None of this occurs without effective leadership at many levels of the organization. This article provides an overview of the principles of leadership, leadership's

Disclosure: The author is a national medical director for Cigna.
Department of Obstetrics and Gynecology, The David Geffen School of Medicine, University of California, Los Angeles, CA, USA
* PO Box 5213, Timonium, MD 21094.
E-mail address: JKeatsMD@gmail.com

role in setting the stage for patient safety, and how these function to enable teams to deliver consistently safe care over long periods of time.

PRINCIPLES OF LEADERSHIP

Every physician is a leader at some level.[2] In clinical practice, by dint of training and experience, physicians are regarded as leaders by their patients. This remains true even in this era of patient-centricity and shared decision making. But physicians are also leaders in every work setting. A physician in solo practice is the leader of his employees. An obstetrician/gynecologist hospitalist in a birth unit at night is the leader of the staff. This leadership continuum carries through to all the physician's roles, from founding partner of a physician group to hospital department chair, from medical director of a multispecialty group to CEO of a large integrated delivery system. There are common characteristics needed to be a successful leader irrespective of the setting.

President Eisenhower once said "…by leadership we mean the art of getting someone else to do something that you want done because he wants to do it…."[3] Nowhere is that more applicable than in providing safe health care. Leadership in health care, in all settings, requires making patient safety the central focus of daily work. This requires creating a model of leadership, a vision, and a culture.[4]

A Model of Leadership

Traditionally, leaders of health care professionals have been perceived as protecting the autonomy of those they lead while shielding them from outside forces that want them to change behaviors. Additionally, leaders are viewed as being responsible for obtaining ever-increasing shares of scarce resources, such as reimbursements, equipment, operating room time, or time off. The patients played no direct role in this narrow view of health care leadership.

Patient safety demands a different model of leadership. In this view, the leader becomes the patient's advocate. This may conflict with previously perceived entitlements. The leader must model this new behavior personally, and set clear expectations for others. This requires consistent and repeated communication with all team members. Every team member must be accountable for this vision. Over time, adherence to this new model of leadership leads to culture change, essential for sustainability.

Culture Change

Organizational culture is a set of shared values and beliefs that interact with the organization's structure and control systems to produce behavioral norms.[5] "Values and beliefs" are what people think is important. "Structure and control systems" are how things work. "Behavioral norms" are the way things are done. Thus, the way things are done is the result of beliefs applied to work processes. Change and improvement in an organization cannot be accomplished if it runs counter to the prevailing culture. "Culture eats strategy for lunch every day."[6] If patient safety is not considered important to the organization, or if existing processes of care run counter to best safety practices, nothing will improve that organization's performance.

Achieving culture change in an organization is a daunting and slow endeavor. Critical to culture change is changing the physician compact.[4] Traditionally physicians were expected to treat patients and provide high-quality care as defined by each individual physician based on their own training, experience, and preferences. Patient safety and the needs of individual patients were secondary to physicians' expectation of autonomy, access to resources, and protection from imposed changes. To improve the culture of a health care organization requires that physicians and their leaders adopt a new physician compact that puts patients and safety first. In this construct, physicians must collaborate in determining standardized best practices, adhere to those practices, and be accountable for patient-centric care. What they receive in return is input into organizational decisions either directly or through their leaders. By delivering safe, high-quality care they achieve a competitive advantage that can improve compensation and resource availability. This transition to a new physician compact enabling culture change requires leaders to inspire others through vision.

Vision

Motivating individuals is critical to successful leadership. The leader makes the invisible visible.[7] Much of the work around improving patient safety in complex environments involves changing processes of care that are not producing the desired results. Changing processes of care almost always requires changing individuals' behaviors. People by nature have different tolerances for change. For many people, change is associated with a high degree of anxiety. Invariably change is perceived as a loss by someone.[8] To counter this, leaders have to change people's mindset such that dissatisfaction with the status quo and potential improvement outweighs the anxiety and perceived loss caused by change.

Creating a vision of improvement is a powerful way for leaders to get people motivated to change. This is part of the "pull" strategy of change management.[9] Leaders need to develop and nurture the mental image of change promoting enhanced patient safety and work satisfaction. Story-telling is a particularly effective way of communicating such vision.[10] Equally important is conveying this vision through multiple approaches, such as one-on-one discussions, group presentations, individual emails, group mailings, and workplace dashboards. Frequently and consistently conveying the advantages of behavioral change facilitates engagement for changes in organizational culture.

The counterpart to a vision-based "pull" strategy is a "push" strategy known as the "burning platform."[11] This image implies that the current state is intolerable and must change. Unfortunately, in obstetrics/gynecology this often results from one or more instances of patient harm. A push strategy is a useful way to create a sense of urgency around changing behaviors to improve safety. Any change management effort without a sense of urgency is doomed to fail.[12] Often the pace of change in patient safety projects is improved when both strategies are used simultaneously.

Setting Direction

Leaders are expected to set the direction of the organization around clearly communicated goals. As a cadet at West Point, Douglas MacArthur was asked how he would erect a flagpole given a group of men and list of materials. As his fellow cadets wrote furiously, the young MacArthur wrote three words: "Sergeant, erect flagpole."[13] What he understood is that the leader's role is to set a goal and then be willing to delegate the action plan to others.

Health care and patient safety is not as simple as erecting a flagpole. However, a useful construct is to make SMART goals (Specific, Measurable, Achievable, Relevant, and Time-bound) (**Box 1**).[14] This markedly increases the chance for success. "Specific" goals should be stated in narrow terms. "Improving fetal outcomes" is not specific; reducing the percentage of term newborns with a 5-minute Apgar of less than seven, however, is. A measurable goal generally follows from specificity.

Box 1
SMART goals
S = Specific
M = Measurable
A = Achievable
R = Relevant
T = Time-bound
Data from Doran GT. There's a S.M.A.R.T. way to write management's goals and objectives. Management review. AMA Forum 1981;70(11):35–6.

In the example just given, "improving" is not measurable but a percentage is. Next the goal should be achievable. Reducing your birthing unit's primary cesarean rate to 10% is almost certainly not achievable (or safe) and will be perceived as futile. Setting an unrealistic goal discourages participation, and often leads to half-hearted implementation. Reducing the primary cesarean rate to the 23.9% recommended by Healthy People 2020 may be perceived as more attainable. People generally care about attaining relevant goals. Reducing the incidence of low Apgar scores is something everyone should care about. Setting a goal of increasing the number of new mothers who go home on the first postpartum day may be relevant to hospital financial officers but probably not to clinical staff. Lastly there must be a specific timeframe to accomplish the goal. Failure to make a goal time-bound invites everyone to put other more time-sensitive tasks ahead of it.

A classic example of successful application of these principles was the Institute for Healthcare Improvement's 100,00 Lives Campaign.[15] Its official motto was "Some is not a number, soon is not a time." Starting in January 2005 it set a goal of reducing hospital mortality nationally by 100,000 in 18 months through the institution of six specific evidence-based measures. These included safety bundles related to ventilator associated pneumonia, central line infections, and the establishment of rapid response teams. The program fulfilled all the requirements of a SMART goal. Ultimately, more than three-fourths (3100) of the hospitals in the United States participated demonstrating its relevance. Although some were skeptical, in June 2006 Institute for Healthcare Improvement announced that 122,000 deaths were prevented. This success led to a Five Million Lives campaign to reduce incidences of harm and replication of this program in many other countries.[16]

People Management Skills

To be an effective leader, one has to be able to manage the people who report to you or look to you for guidance and direction. A leader must first understand his or her own emotional intelligence.[17] Emotional intelligence as a leader involves self-awareness and social-awareness. Self-awareness involves understanding your moods, emotions, and drives, and how to maximize your strengths and minimize your weaknesses. Doing this improves how you are perceived by others and impacts their willingness to follow your directions and imperatives. Social awareness refers to building relationships with others through empathy and motivation toward achieving a common goal. There is no correlation between high academic achievement and emotional intelligence.[17] Successful leaders tend to be self-aware and socially aware. Emotional intelligence is a stronger indicator of success in leadership than other measures of intelligence.

How can you use your emotional intelligence to improve performance by those you lead? One way is to "catch people doing something right."[18] Excellent leaders know that positive feedback about something done well goes a long way to keep morale high and motivate people to work hard. This positive feedback can be brief, consisting of a few words, a hand shake, or literal pat on the back, or it can be a small material token of appreciation. Recognition does not have to elaborate or be done in front of a group. The key thing is timing. This is most effective when done proximate to the good performance, that is, "catching" people doing the right thing. Rewarding and celebrating intermediate successes is an important principle of change management.[12] If your goal is to increase participation in departmental drills and simulations by 50% in 6 months, recognizing progress made toward that goal at 2 and 4 months helps sustain the efforts. These "progress reports" keep everyone focused and motivated. It also creates peer pressure for everyone to engage with the effort.

Involve All Stakeholders

When trying to improve the safety of care in any setting, it is necessary to develop a strategy through changing work processes. When deciding what to change and how to change it, deliberations must involve everyone affected.[19] In the setting of a labor unit, for example, this includes not just the physicians, midwives, and nurses, but potentially the unit secretaries, the environmental services workers, the pharmacists, the unit volunteers, and a patient advocate. The goal is to prevent the "not invented here phenomenon." Any change process that you design and implement will be at best resisted and at worst sabotaged by any group that was not included in formulating the change. "Men often oppose a thing merely because they have had no agency in planning it, or because it may have been planned by those whom they dislike."[20]

Part of the problem with involving all stakeholders in designing a change process is in the very act of bringing people. When people from different disciplines and job descriptions are brought together to problem solve, the perceived hierarchy inhibits some people from speaking up. Nurses may be hesitant to voice ideas in front of physicians, whereas unit secretaries may feel inhibited from contributing to a discussion at all. Invariably even within disciplines there may be one or two individuals who attempt to dominate the discussion. Others may have better solutions but are reluctant to speak up. An effective way to engage everyone uses the nominal group technique (**Box 2**).[21]

In nominal group technique the leader presents a clear statement of the problem. Each participant is then given time to silently and individually write down as many

---

Box 2
Nominal group technique

- Individual team members silently brainstorm and capture their ideas.

- All ideas are captured through a round-robin recording of ideas.

- Each idea is briefly discussed for clarification and understanding. Similar ideas are grouped or combined.

- Each team member selects the top 3 to 5 ideas he or she thinks is most important and ranks them. The rankings of all team members are combined and summed.

Reprinted with permission from Tague NR. The Quality Toolbox, Second Edition. Milwaukee: ASQ Quality Press © 2005 ASQ, www.asq.org. All rights reserved.

possible solutions that they can think of. The leader then goes around the room calling on every participant to state one solution. These are captured on a flip chart without questions or discussion. Anyone who has thought of the same solution crosses it off their list. This continues around the room as many times as necessary until every idea is captured. Once that is complete, clarifying questions are asked of the author of any suggestion, and similar suggestions are grouped together. Several potential solutions are thus posited. The group then silently votes for the top five solutions based on their perception of feasibility and likelihood for success. The best solution is given a score of five, the next best four, and so forth. The score sheets are then collected and tallied by the leader in front of the group. The highest scoring solutions then become the consensus of the group as to how the organization will proceed. This technique is a great way to not only arrive at a solution that otherwise may have gone unvoiced, but also to get critical buy-in from all parties. This greatly enhances the likelihood that everyone will support the change process.

Standardization

Standardization of care processes is the last leadership tool to reduce error and prevent harm. Standardization of care, through the use of clinical guidelines and checklists, has been shown to reduce patient harm in multiple clinical settings.[22] Reducing variation in the administration of potentially harmful drugs, such as oxytocin and magnesium sulfate, reduces the chance of human error. The challenge for leaders often is to convince a group of physicians who value clinical autonomy to embrace standardization.

It is important to distinguish two types of clinical variation: necessary and unexplained. Necessary clinical variation is determined by characteristics inherent in an individual patient. Unexplained clinical variation is determined by differences in how physicians approach similar patients based on their own experiences, training, and sometimes biases. Standardization seeks to eliminate these unexplained clinical variations.

Standardization is a difficult concept for physicians, most of whom are convinced that they know the one "right" way to do almost anything. This leads to unexplained clinical variation. For example, there has never been a study to demonstrate the single best regimen for oxytocin administration for induction or augmentation of labor. In a large obstetric department, lack of standardization can lead to multiple different regimens. This in turn increases the risk of nursing error, tachysystole, and fetal distress. Instead, choosing a single departmental oxytocin regimen avoids those issues. The physician may always alter the protocol for an individual patient if necessary. They must, however, document in the patient's chart the clinical reasoning behind the deviation. These episodes are then reviewed for validity. Frequent deviations would indicate a need to review and possibly modify the protocol. In this iterative way, any clinical protocol becomes a dynamic document. The department develops a standard "best practice" for administering oxytocin in most patients. In this way, leaders implement standardization as a pathway to providing safe, high-quality care.

PRINCIPLES OF TEAMWORK

One cannot provide patient care alone. The sheer complexity of modern medical care demands that care for most patients be delivered in teams. There are several foundational concepts that allow health care teams to function with maximal efficiency and safety. Application of these concepts to every care setting facilitates implementation of goals at the point of patient care.

Communication

The heart of teamwork is communication. Unless messages are clearly sent and received, teams cannot function. The Joint Commission estimated that in 72% of neonatal injury or death cases, communication failure was a contributing factor.[23] Patient safety leaders must ensure unambiguous communication, critical for highly functioning patient care teams.

There are multiple tools and techniques to improve team communication. One goal is overcoming hesitancy to speak because of hierarchies even when a problem is observed. A series of wrong-site and wrong-procedure surgeries at an academic medical center was related to operating room nurses not speaking up because they feared retribution.[24] Developed by the airline industry in response to several major accidents, Crew Resource Management seeks to flatten hierarchies and facilitates everyone on the team speaking up when there is a perceived safety threat.[25] This is especially useful in operating room or labor units, similar to a commercial airline crew, where individuals not always familiar with each other are expected to perform highly complex tasks safely. In a busy obstetric unit, with dozens of nurses, physicians, scrub technicians, surgical assistants, and others, there are thousands of combinations of participants that might form a team for a cesarean birth. The expectation is that anyone will speak up if they have a safety concern. Simply having every participant introduce themselves and their role before the start of surgery encourages communication and speaking up if necessary, thereby reducing patient harm.[26] Drills and simulations (See Jean-Ju Sheen and Dena Goffman's article, "Emerging Role of Drills and Simulations in Patient Safety," in this issue.) further improve team communication in emergencies.

Lastly, structured communications improve accuracy and completeness. One commonly used technique is SBAR (Situation, Background, Assessment, Recommendation/request) communication (**Box 3**).[27] SBAR gives the recipient the background to focus on a clinical issue with a clear set of recommendations from the sender for further action. There should be the opportunity for discussion to clarify any ambiguous items. TeamSTEPPS program from the Agency for Healthcare Research and Quality incorporates other communication tools, such as CUS (Concerned, Uncomfortable, Scared) to clearly convey the gravity of the safety issue and demand attention.[28] This then helps the leader take the appropriate action ranging from investigating the issue to "stopping the line." Another example is the Two-Challenge Rule. If a team

---

Box 3
SBAR

S – Situation: What is the clinical event or change in status that is prompting the communication?

B – Background: What are the relevant parts of the patient's history that may help arrive at an appropriate response?

A – Assessment: What does the initiator of the communication believe is the problem or is concerned may be the problem?

R - Recommendation/request: What action would the initiator of the communication like the recipient to take?

Data from American College of Obstetricians and Gynecologists Committee on Patient Safety and Quality Improvement. Committee Opinion No. 590: preparing for clinical emergencies in obstetrics and gynecology. Obstet Gynecol 2014;123(3):722–5.

member's safety concern is not satisfactorily addressed, they should raise it again. An inadequate response should empower the individual to use the chain of command until they receive appropriate explanations or corrective actions.

Situational Awareness

Situational awareness defined as "the perception of environmental elements and events with respect to time or space, the comprehension of their meaning, and the projection of their future status" is a critical team asset.[29] Situational awareness should always be able to answer three questions:

1. What is happening now?
2. What do we expect to happen in the next hour, day, etc.?
3. What are we going to do if #2 does not happen?

For example, answers to these questions for a deteriorating fetal heart rate tracing might be as follows:

1. The fetal heart rate is showing minimal variability and repetitive deep variable decelerations. The patient is remote from delivery. We are administering maternal oxygen, repositioning, increasing intravenous fluids, and starting an amnioinfusion.
2. We expect the fetal heart rate tracing to improve in the next 30 minutes, with improved variability and cessation of the decelerations.
3. If the tracing is not improved in 30 minutes we will move the patient to the operating room and prepare for a cesarean birth.

Part of team situational awareness is a shared mental model of the current and expected status of all the patients under the team's care. This is achieved through huddles. Huddles may occur at preset times during which the team reviews the status of all of their patients or may be initiated anytime a team member needs to alert everyone about a significant change in a patient's status.[30] In a labor unit, this is most often done at nursing shift changes. Ideally all disciplines, including obstetrics, anesthesia, neonatal intensive care unit/pediatrics, and nursing, gather in a central place to update everyone on the status of every patient. Even in busy units this is accomplished in a short amount of time. This information exchanged improves team function. It also helps anticipate the need for additional resources and personnel.

Team Learning

Highly functioning teams strive to improve performance by continuous learning.[31] To achieve this goal, drills and simulations have become more common.

Debriefing is another strategy to promote team learning and improve performance. Debriefing brings together of all participants to review everyone's actions at the conclusion of an incident.[32] These events are opportunities for team learning from what went well and where improvement is needed. Debriefing is the start of that process. It should occur soon after the event, while everyone's memories are fresh. It should occur even if a mistake did not cause patient harm, a "near miss." These cases of "near misses" may be especially helpful to learn what prevented an error from causing harm.

Debriefings should follow a set format. A printed form helps the leader follow this format and record information that facilitates team learning. The discussion should always be nonjudgmental. A typical format for a debriefing is as follows:

1. What went well? The team should acknowledge what standardized procedures were correctly followed, perhaps as previously rehearsed in mock drills. Excellent performance by individual members should be called out.

2. What did not go well? The team identifies areas where individual or team performance was suboptimal. These areas may become the focus for future simulations. Often, this discussion identifies system deficiencies. Was a key to a locked medicine cabinet not available? Was the automated medication dispenser not stocked, was critical equipment not in place?

3. What are we going to do differently next time? How will the standard protocol for this particular event be revised to allow better, more rapid response to a crisis? In what areas does the team need additional training? How can we communicate better during an emergency?

4. Who are we going to tell? It is vital that the team leader communicate system deficiencies to someone with the authority to correct them. The leader then needs to "close the loop" by reporting corrective action back to the team.

5. Is everyone OK? In the event of patient harm, individuals on the team will harbor guilt feelings and may suffer a form of post-traumatic stress syndrome.[33] Whether justified or not, they may blame themselves for the outcome. Recognizing this possibility, and identifying team members who harbor such feelings, is an important role of team leaders. These vulnerable team members may need counseling or therapy.

Information from a debrief must be transmitted to those in the organization responsible for quality improvement. An individual must be responsible for investigating and correcting the deficiencies identified. Appropriate systems solutions must be developed to reduce the risk for reoccurrence. Attention should be given to providers traumatized by incidents of patient harm. Lessons learned from a case thus improve care throughout the system.

SUMMARY

Leadership and teamwork are two sides a single coin. One cannot be a leader without followers in the form of a team, and a team cannot function optimally without leadership. Obstetricians/gynecologists work in some of the most complex care environments. Providing consistently safe care in these settings is a challenge that requires constant attention. It requires leaders who can create a vision of standardized, evidence-based care delivered in a culture where patient safety is everyone's responsibility. It is also a culture where teamwork is highly valued, and emergency scenarios are rehearsed through drills and simulations. It is a culture where excellent communication skills promote situational awareness and team learning. It is a culture where the best care is delivered reliably; where the satisfaction of the patients, their families, and the caregivers themselves is prized above everything else. This should be the goal of every health care provider in every practice setting. It can be achieved through the application of the principles of leadership and teamwork.

REFERENCES

1. Chantler C. The role and education of doctors in the delivery of health care. Lancet 1999;353(9159):1178–81.

2. Kwon E, Flood P. Physician leadership lessons from the business world. Fam Pract Manag 2016;23(6):14–6. Available at: https://www.aafp.org/fpm/2016/1100/p14.html. Accessed October 17, 2018.

3. Dwight David Eisenhower: remarks at the annual conference of the society for personnel administration. Available at: http://www.presidency.ucsb.edu/ws/index.php?pid=9884. Accessed October 17, 2018.

4. Silvers J, Kornacki MJ. Leading physicians through change: how to achieve and sustain results. Tampa (FL): American College of Physician Executives; 2012.

5. Groysberg B, Lee J, Price J, et al. The leader's guide to corporate culture Harvard business review 2018. Available at: https://hbr.org/2018/01/the-culture-factor. Accessed November 5, 2018.

6. Campbell D, Edgar D, Storehouse G. Business strategy: an introduction. 3rd edition. London: Palgrave Macmillan; 2011. p. 263.

7. Thatchenkery T, Sugiyama K. Making the invisible visible. London: Palgrave Macmillan; 2011.

8. Connelly M. Kubler-Ross five stage model. Available at: https://www.change-management-coach.com/kubler-ross.html access. Accessed November 5, 2018.

9. Boive CA. Change management: deciding whether to push or pull. Available at: https://www.itbusiness.ca/blog/change-management-deciding-whether-to-push-or-pull/31268. Accessed November 5, 2018.

10. Jacoby J. Use storytelling technique to communicate your vision. Available at: https://www.leadersbeacon.com/how-to-use-storytelling-technique-to-communicate-your-vision/. Accessed November 5, 2018.

11. Anthony SD. How to anticipate a burning platform. Harvard Business Review. Available at: https://hbr.org/2012/12/how-to-anticipate-a-burning-platform. Accessed November 5, 2018.

12. Kotter JP. Leading change. Boston: Harvard Business Review Press; 2012.

13. Sailer S. Memorium - Jerry Pournelle Taki's Magazine 2017. Available at: http://takimag.com/article/in_memoriam_jerry_pournelle/print#ixzz5UCO0xl8A. Accessed October 28, 2018.

14. Doran GT. There's a S.M.A.R.T. way to write management's goals and objectives. Management Review. AMA Forum 1981;70(11):35–6. Available at: https://community.mis.temple.edu/mis0855002fall2015/files/2015/10/S.M.A.R.T-Way-Management-Review.pdf.

15. Berwick DM, Calkins DR, McCannon CJ, et al. The 100,000 lives campaign: setting a goal and a deadline for improving health care quality. J Am Med Assoc 2006;295(3):324–7.

16. Berwick DM. Promising care: how we can rescue health care by improving it. "Chapter 2: some is not a number, soon is not a time. San Francisco (CA): Jossey-Bass; 2014.

17. Coleman D. Emotional intelligence. New York: Bantam Books; 1995.

18. Blanchard K, Johnson S. The one minute manager. New York: William Morrow and Co; 1982.

19. Ajaz M. Why identification of stakeholders is important in project management. Available at: https://www.linkedin.com/pulse/why-identification-stakeholders-important-project-mohammed-ajaz-pmp/. Accessed November 5, 2018.

20. Hamilton A. The Federalist Papers no. 70. Available at: http://avalon.law.yale.edu/18th_century/fed70.asp. Accessed November 5, 2018.

21. Tague NR. The quality toolbox. 2nd edition. Milwaukee (WI): ASQ Quality Press; 2004. p. 364–5.

22. Committee on Patient Safety and Quality Improvement. Committee opinion no. 629: clinical guidelines and standardization of practice to improve outcomes. Obstet Gynecol 2015;125:1027–9.

23. The Joint Commission: Sentinel event alert issue #30 - Preventing infant death and injury during delivery July 21. Available at: https://www.jointcommission.org/assets/1/18/SEA_30.PDF. Accessed November 6, 2018.

24. Duhigg C. The power of habit. Chapter Five. New York: Random House; 2012.

25. McConaughey E. Crew resource management in healthcare: the evolution of teamwork training and medteams. J Perinat Neonatal Nurs 2008;22(2):96–104.
26. Committee Opinion No. 464. Patient safety in the surgical environment. Obstet Gynecol 2010;116:786–90.
27. American College of Obstetricians and Gynecologists Committee on Patient Safety and Quality Improvement. Committee Opinion No. 590. Preparing for clinical emergencies in obstetrics and gynecology. Obstet Gynecol 2014;123: 722–5.
28. Agency for Healthcare Research and Quality. TeamSTEPPS: national implementation. Available at: http://teamstepps.ahrq.gov/abouttoolsmaterials.htm. Accessed November 6, 2018.
29. Schulz CM, Endsley MR, Kochs EF, et al. Situation awareness in anesthesia: concept and research. Anesthesiology 2013;118(3):729–42.
30. Institute for Healthcare Improvement: daily huddles. Available at: http://www.ihi.org/resources/Pages/Tools/Huddles.aspx. Accessed November 6, 2018.
31. Bendaly L, Bendaly N. Improving healthcare team performance. Hoboken (NJ): Josses-Bass; 2012.
32. Agency for Healthcare Research and Quality Patient Safety Primer. Debriefing for clinical learning. Available at: https://psnet.ahrq.gov/primers/primer/36/Debriefing-for-Clinical-Learning. Accessed November 6, 2018.
33. Wu A. Medical error: the second victim. BMJ 2000;320:726.

Emerging Role of Drills and Simulations in Patient Safety

Jean-Ju Sheen, MD, Dena Goffman, MD*

KEYWORDS

- Drills and simulations in obstetrics • Drills and simulations in gynecology
- Drills and simulations in patient safety in obstetrics
- Drills and simulations in patient safety in gynecology

KEY POINTS

- Ensuring patient safety and optimizing outcomes in obstetrics and gynecology through improving technical skills, enhancing team performance, and decreasing medical errors has resulted in significant interest in incorporating drills and simulation into medical training, continuing education, and multidisciplinary team practice.
- Drills and simulations are ideal because of their wide range of application with various learners and settings.
- Drills and simulations provide a safe space to learn and maintain technical skills and to improve knowledge, confidence, communication, and teamwork behaviors, particularly for less common, high-stakes clinical scenarios.

INTRODUCTION

The concept of promoting patient safety by preventing medical errors is not new. In the early 1900s, patient safety pioneer and surgeon Ernest Amory Codman, MD (1869–1940) linked medical care, preventable errors, and outcomes, yet his efforts "brought him mostly ridicule, poverty, and censure."[1] Despite additional research that continued to document frequent episodes of preventable harm in hospitalized patients, safety in medicine remained underdeveloped until the 1990s.[2] The landmark Institute of Medicine report, *To Err Is Human*, with its estimation that 44,000 to 98,000 Americans die each year due to preventable harm, spurred the beginning of the modern patient safety movement.[2,3] Although there has been great variation in the numbers quoted, this and subsequent publications sparked renewed attention to improving patient safety in

Disclosure Statement: The authors report no commercial or financial conflicts of interest.
Department of Obstetrics and Gynecology, Columbia University Irving Medical Center, 622 West 168th Street PH 16, New York, NY 10032, USA
* Corresponding author.
E-mail address: dg2018@cumc.columbia.edu

hospitals and other health care settings, bringing both increased understanding of the root causes of safety issues and progress in decreasing preventable harm, while secondarily reducing the burdensome cost of medical care.[2,4]

Contemporaneous to the growing movement toward decreasing medical errors was the restricted duty hour standards set in 2003 by the Accreditation Council for Graduate Medical Education, for all accredited medical training institutions in the United States.[5] This well-intentioned attempt at preventing overtired physicians from making critical medical decisions may have resulted in other unforeseen adverse safety consequences. Work-hour reductions pose additional challenges to ensuring adequate clinical experience for obstetrics and gynecology trainees, who require broad exposure to increasingly complex procedures, diagnoses, clinical emergencies, and their management. Educators, seeking innovative methods to teach dwindling skills resulting from this decreased exposure to clinical medicine, are turning to the use of drills and simulation. Because of their versatility, drills and simulations are ideal for teaching and retaining skills for basic procedures (such as cervical examinations) to complex, rarely encountered obstetrics and gynecologic emergencies (such as malignant hyperthermia) while uncovering latent systems issues.

Simulations and drills are becoming increasingly used for experienced clinicians and teams in addition to trainees. Practicing critical technical skills for managing rare events, like shoulder dystocia, benefits even the most experienced clinicians. Perhaps most importantly, simulation affords the opportunity to identify potential failures in teamwork and communication, which are consistently cited as contributors to adverse events. Reviewing these skills in a safe place helps with implementation of new best practices and identification of latent issues that can be corrected before harm to a patient.

DRILLS AND SIMULATIONS DEFINED

Drills and simulations are terms often used together in the medical education literature. Although they both have an important role in improving patient safety and outcomes, their applications and specific goals are distinct, even if they are used in concert with each other. A drill is practice involving repetition of an activity in order to improve a skill, or a particular occasion for such practice.[6] Drills may lead to improved standardization of response, provider satisfaction, and patient outcomes.[7] Examples of drills include training for operative vaginal deliveries or intrauterine contraceptive device placement.

On the other hand, simulation has been defined as a situation in which a particular set of conditions is created artificially in order to study or experience something that is possible in real life, the artificial representation of a real world process to achieve educational goals via experimental learning.[8] Simulation-based education uses simulators, devices that enable the operator to reproduce or represent under test conditions phenomena likely to occur in actual performance, or other simulative aids to replicate clinical scenarios, serving as alternatives to real patients.[9] Examples of simulated scenarios include management of hypertensive emergencies in obstetrics and gynecology, such as eclamptic seizures on a labor and delivery unit or malignant hypertension in the gynecologic operating room.

THE EVOLUTION OF MEDICAL EDUCATION TOWARD INCORPORATION OF SIMULATION

Medical education evolved during the last century from a simple apprenticeship to the incorporation of learning scientific principles, and, finally, to the requirement of objective measures of competence in the domains of knowledge, skills, and behaviors.[10] Opportunities to fortify skills have decreased, as work-hour limitations have been implemented. Patients have become increasingly concerned that students and physicians in training are "practicing" on them. There is a concern that clinical medicine has become more focused on patient safety and quality than on bedside teaching and education.[11] Undeniably, practice is a basic requirement for learning and maintaining skills, as recognized in many nonmedical fields, such as music.[10] Medical education has only recently applied the concept of deliberate practice to gain and retain medical skills, rendering obsolete the apprentice-style education model of "see one, do one, teach one" in the setting of increasing concern for the quality of patient care and safety, and changes in the health care systems.[9,12]

Although the use of simulations and drills in medical education has gained more recognition in the last few decades, historical evidence indicates they have roots in antiquity, with some applications being quite sophisticated. During the Song Dynasty in China, imperial physician Wang Wei-Yi (987–1067) trained students using life-sized bronze statues containing wooden organs and 354 holes covered in wax and filled with a liquid that would drip after a correctly placed acupuncture needle was removed.[13] Simulation and drills in obstetrics and gynecology also had early historic origins: the mid-eighteenth century surgeon Giovanni Antonio Galli designed a birthing simulator composed of a glass uterus in a pelvis and a flexible fetus, in order to train midwives and surgeons in childbirth.[14]

The increased incorporation of patient simulation and drills toward the end of the twentieth century was a major step in the evolution of health sciences education.[10] Because many students think that they are inadequately trained in history taking, physical examination, diagnosis, and management, these tools have been proposed as a technique to bridge this educational gap between the classroom and clinical environment.[11]

IMPROVING PATIENT SAFETY THROUGH SIMULATION AND DRILLS IN OBSTETRICS AND GYNECOLOGY

Medical simulations and drills have played an increasingly important role in the education of obstetricians and gynecologists throughout their career. In 2007, the American College of Obstetricians and Gynecologists (ACOG) formed 2 task forces, Simulation for Resident Education and On Reentry, recognizing simulation as a valuable education component for graduate and postgraduate education.[15] The subsequent formation of the ACOG Simulation Consortium created simulation-based obstetric and surgical skills training for obstetrics/gynecology residents as an adjunct to traditional procedural-oriented education. This consortium has since evolved to become the ACOG Simulation Working Group, with a current mission to establish simulation as a pillar in education for women's health, through collaboration, advocacy, research, and the development and implementation of multidisciplinary simulations-based educational resources and opportunities for obstetrics and gynecology.

In its Committee Opinion, Patient Safety in Obstetrics and Gynecology, ACOG listed a set of quality and patient safety objectives that should be adopted by obstetrician-gynecologists in their practices[16]:

I. Develop a commitment to encourage a culture of patient safety
II. Implement recommended safe medication practices
III. Reduce the likelihood of surgical errors
IV. Improve communication with health care providers
V. Improve communication with patients

VI. Establish a partnership with patients to improve safety
VII. Make safety a priority in every aspect of practice

Meeting and sustaining these objectives in clinical practice would be more attainable if they were incorporated during an obstetrician/gynecologist's formative years in medical school and postgraduate training and then reinforced during clinical practice. These ACOG patient safety objectives may be met through the routine use of drills and simulations in obstetrics and gynecology education and clinical practice.

A recent PubMed search of the terms "simulation and obstetrics or gynecology" in article titles and abstracts suggests rapid growth in the field of simulation in recent years, yielding 20 articles published in the year 2007 and 175 articles published in 2017. The range of clinical skills and scenarios that have been simulated in obstetrics and gynecology is vast: from specific basic skills such as vaginal delivery and perineal repair in obstetrics and intrauterine contraceptive device placement in gynecology to complex medical scenarios, such as maternal cardiac arrest or management of a major vascular injury during laparoscopic surgery (**Box 1**). Although there is large variation in the types of simulations that can be created, the critical components to crafting a successful simulation are the same for all: identification and involvement of key stakeholders, recruitment and training of capable people to lead the simulations, and perhaps most importantly, identification and prioritization of objectives. Goals should be explicit: clinical knowledge, teamwork, and communication skills should be integrated, process and outcome measures should be delineated, and opportunity for debriefing and feedback should be incorporated into the timeline planned to perform the simulation. The framework for achieving these goals may be set by using the 5 Ws: Who? What? When? Where? Why?, and 2 Hs: How? and How Often?, which may guide the development of a simulation program highly tailored to the team of learners in mind.[15]

WHO?

The learners in both obstetrics and gynecology simulations run the gamut in range of experience, knowledge, and skill. They may include medical students, residents, fellows, attending physicians, nurses, midwives, and midlevel providers. They may include people from varying disciplines, including general obstetrics, maternal-fetal medicine, anesthesia, pediatrics, and critical care (for obstetrics) and general gynecology, anesthesia, gynecologic oncology, and the other surgical subspecialties (for gynecology) The learners may be individuals, or they may be in teams. Anyone involved in the outcome for the patient may be a learner in a simulation. However, a unifying characteristic of these learners is that they are all adults. The most current trainees and young physicians are millennials who have learning styles distinct from their predecessors.

Adult learning provides many challenges that are different from traditional students because their actions are affected by previous life experiences, ingrained personality traits, and relationship patterns.[17,18] Adult learners become more self-directed with time, preferring their learning to be problem centered, meaningful, and immediately applicable.[17,19] Receptiveness toward learning opportunities depends on factors such as their motivation for attending training, whether it is voluntary or mandatory, and whether recertification or job retention requires the learning activity in question.[17] The most current generation of medical students, residents, and junior attendings belong to Generation Y, the millennial generation (born in 1977–1995), whose style of learning is more heavily reliant on technology than in previous generations.[20] Their preferred instruction is technology enhanced, convenient, personalized, and

Box 1
Suggested simulations in obstetrics and gynecology

Obstetrics
  Fetal procedures
    Amniocentesis
    Cordocentesis
    Chorionic villous sampling
    Fetal shunt placement
  Labor management
    Cervical examination
    Artificial rupture of membranes
    Placement of intrauterine pressure
    Catheter
    Placement of fetal scalp electrode
  Vaginal deliveries
    Cephalic delivery
    Breech delivery
    Shoulder dystocia
    Operative vaginal delivery
    Perineal/laceration repair
  Cesarean deliveries
    Hemorrhage
    Cesarean section
    Umbilical cord prolapse
  Critical care obstetrics
    Hypertensive urgency/eclampsia
    Sepsis
    Cardiac arrest
    Diabetic ketoacidosis
    Thyroid storm
    Hemorrhage

Neonatal procedures
  Neonatal resuscitation
  Circumcision

Communication skills
  Breaking bad news
  Apology and disclosure
  Difficult conversations
  Informed consent
  Deposition

Gynecology
  Office procedures
    Long-acting reversible
    Contraceptive placement
    Endometrial biopsy
    Bartholin gland cyst/abscess
    Incision and drainage
    Placement of Word catheter
  Vaginal procedures
    Cold-knife cone biopsy
    Urologic sling placement
    Uterine aspiration
    Anterior vaginal wall dissection
    Vaginal hysterectomy
  Laparoscopy
    Ovarian cystectomy
    Tubal sterilization
    Salpingectomy

Hysteroscopy
Laparotomy
   Abdominal hysterectomy
   Pelvic sidewall dissection
Cystoscopy
Intraoperative emergencies
   Malignant hyperthermia
   Subcutaneous emphysema
   Hemorrhage
   Adverse anesthetic reaction
   Fire in the operating room
   Disaster or mass casualty

relevant.[21] Because simulations and drills tend to be interactive and hands-on, they appeal to millennial learners. Traditional unidirectional teaching methods (ie, didactic teaching facts to students) are ineffective in adult learning and may be even less useful in team training exercises.[17] The estimated half-life of professional knowledge from formal education may be as short as 2 to 2.5 years.[22] If an activity requires both knowledge and a core skill set, such as Advanced Cardiac Life Support, retention can be as short as 6 to 12 months.[23,24]

In recognizing the nature of adult learners and their generational context, those setting up drills or simulation exercises can maximize their effectiveness and skill retention by picking high-yield, relevant topics and appropriate intervals of time between exercises for reinforcement.

WHAT?

The utility of simulation as a tool in obstetrics and gynecology lies in its seemingly limitless range of application (see **Box 1**). Simulation allows the trainee to gain facility in obstetric technical maneuvers, such as a simple normal spontaneous cephalic delivery, to the more complicated breech and operative vaginal deliveries, to emergency situations, such as shoulder dystocia. For higher-level education promoting knowledge and its application, one may simulate more extended scenarios, such as postpartum hemorrhage, eclampsia, and maternal cardiac arrest, using high-fidelity mannequins.

In gynecology, basic surgical skills and technical outpatient office skills (placement of long-acting reversible contraception, such as intrauterine devices or implantable hormones) and endoscopic skills (laparoscopy, hysteroscopy) may be simulated using simple task-trainers or more advanced technology, such as virtual reality. Although there have been fewer simulations in the field of gynecology, the literature has been growing steadily. More complex skills (such as hysterectomy and pelvic sidewall dissection) are particularly important to simulate because of decreasing opportunities to perform open abdominal cases due to rising trends toward performing minimally invasive surgeries. Some of the critical care issues in obstetrics also lend themselves to simulations in gynecology, such as massive hemorrhage and cardiac arrest, and the knowledge gleaned from these simulations has applicability to both fields.

WHEN AND WHERE?

Education through drills and simulations may be performed almost any time and place, but generally there are 3 broad categories for timing (during dedicated teaching time, scheduled simulation time, unannounced drills) and 2 broad categories for location (in situ or not in situ, such as in a simulation center). The ideal program is likely to use a combination of these categories to accomplish different learning objectives. Advantages and disadvantages exist for each approach.

The use of dedicated teaching time has the advantage of allowing teaching in a more innovative and learner-centered way due to advanced scheduling and planning. Adding additional scheduled simulation time can afford these benefits but may place a burden on calendars. Alternatively, unannounced in situ drills and simulations have the advantages of a more realistic feel, the presence of the real-life team, the capability of identifying real systems issues, and decreased cost. However, the disadvantages include the challenges for teams due to competing clinical priorities. Staff may feel obliged to care for their "real" patients during their simulations and may be unable to immerse themselves fully in the learning opportunity. Use of clinical spaces may impede patient flow and take away resources needed from patients and staff not involved in the simulation. These drills may often need to be moved, postponed, or canceled depending on real patient volume and acuity.

Simulation center experiences have the advantages of allowing for a dedicated time and place without the potential distractions from clinical duties. Participants may feel more protected and have less performance anxiety because there may be fewer observers. Disadvantages include the difficulty of achieving the "suspension of disbelief" that is critical for a successful simulation or drill. Real systems issues may be overlooked because of differences in the simulation center compared with in situ clinical spaces.

Although each category has advantages and disadvantages, studies have shown that knowledge and performance improve after simulation training regardless of the location of the training.[25,26] Ultimately the choice of site and timing needs to be individualized to the capability of the institution performing the simulation or drill. The flexibility and adaptability of these tools are a major benefit to incorporating them into patient safety and outcomes improvement initiatives.

HOW AND HOW OFTEN?

The types of simulators used for both obstetrics and gynecology are as varied as the scenarios they portray. Simulators range from low technology to high fidelity, with ranges of prices to match. In addition, the use of patient actors can add to the scenario by helping participants to work on communicating with the simulated patient and can contribute to participant ability to "suspend disbelief," which can enhance the authenticity of the exercise. One study demonstrated that regardless of fidelity of the model used, all simulation training improved learners' management of shoulder dystocia, but more successful deliveries were achieved with less force when a high-fidelity training mannequin was used.[27] In obstetric emergency training, all interdisciplinary training improved patient-actor perception of care. Training with a patient actor may improve the perception of safety and communication more than training with a high-fidelity mannequin.[28]

How often to repeat simulation training may depend on the frequency of occurrence of the clinical situation in real life, in addition to its medical complexity and level of learner involved. Following baseline evaluation and shoulder dystocia simulation training, skill retention was evaluated at 3, 6, and 12 months. Croft and colleagues[29] found that these skills were maintained for at least 1 year.

WHY?

The benefits of drills and simulations for individual learners, teams, patients, and institutions are innumerable. The set of lessons gleaned from root cause analyses has been consistent in demonstrating failures resulting in safety lapses of which can be addressed with well-designed simulation experiences. Recurrent themes identified include the failure to recognize an unsafe situation, the failure to seek senior input, poor teamwork, inadequate skill of the team, and poor communication. Maslovitz and colleagues[30] studied labor and delivery teams dealing with simulated emergencies, demonstrating that the most common management errors were delay in transporting the bleeding patient to the operating room, unfamiliarity with prostaglandin administration to reverse uterine atony, delayed blood transfusion to reverse consumption coagulopathy, poor cardiopulmonary resuscitation techniques, inadequate documentation of shoulder dystocia, and inappropriate avoidance of episiotomy in shoulder dystocia and breech extraction. When a portion of the trainees were invited for repeated sessions at least 6 months after the first training day, their performances were significantly improved.[30]

Drills and simulations provide a safe environment where learners have a "hands-on" experience during which they can make mistakes without consequence. The scenarios can range from common to rare and simple to complex, providing opportunities that otherwise might first be encountered when treating a critically ill patient. Literature in both medical and nonmedical fields suggests 5000 or more hours of deliberate learning and practice or 10 years of intense experience is necessary to become an expert and achieve a high level of competency.[12] With work-hour duty restrictions and shifts in the volumes of types of procedures performed, drills and simulations can help increase learning opportunities for achieving adequate competency, especially for low-volume procedures and critical care management.

Besides the benefits gained by the individual learner, drills and simulations also provide a unique opportunity for team-training and improvement of communication skills, with the flexibility of accommodating varying numbers of participants. Scenarios may be designed to have specific objectives tailored to each individual or team involved, in addition to having more global objectives, such as establishing care standards. Both individuals and teams would have the opportunity to reflect on their performance during debriefings sessions, which would serve to reinforce desired skills and behaviors.

For a truly comprehensive patient safety program, all potential causes of harm should be elucidated and remedied, if possible. In significant safety events, root cause analyses often uncover system issues that contribute to the adverse outcomes. Drills and simulations allow for the evaluation of systems before an adverse event so that concerning issues may be discovered and remedied in a proactive way before impacting a patient.

Multiple studies have demonstrated improved learner performance in the simulated environment after simulation training. There is now ample evidence in the obstetrics literature that simulation training also improves patient care, safety, and outcomes. Crofts and colleagues[31] investigated the management and outcomes of shoulder dystocia in the 12 years following implementation of shoulder dystocia training. They found that continued training improved compliance with national guidelines and also significantly decreased neonatal morbidity associated with shoulder dystocia deliveries. Siassakos and colleagues[32] showed that implementation of multidisciplinary training for umbilical cord prolapse was associated with improvements in management, particularly the diagnosis-to-delivery interval.

In the gynecology literature, there are fewer studies evaluating the impact of simulation training on patient care. These gynecologic studies suggest improved outcomes from simulation training, although more studies are needed. Asoğlu and colleagues[33] showed a significant improvement in blood loss before and after simulation-based training for total abdominal and robot-assisted hysterectomies, although no difference was found for total laparoscopic and vaginal hysterectomies.

Last, the use of drills and simulation may increase the public trust of the medical field. With improved efforts to fortify individual and group clinical skills and to enhance teamwork, patients may feel more comfortable knowing their medical team is experienced and is not using them for purposes of "practice."

There are a multitude of ways to incorporate drills and simulation into obstetrics and gynecology training programs and postgraduate education. Growing evidence demonstrates that providing these learning opportunities contributes to improved quality and patient safety. By training medical students with this type of hands-on, adult-learning–focused programs, they will enter their professional medical career with an enhanced skill set and readiness to continue learning. In addition, they can use this experience to become better teachers. As these modalities are incorporated into a robust curriculum to standardize exposure and instruction in technical skills, communication, and complex clinical management, residents and fellows will complete their training demonstrating skills in key elements before going out into practice. For trainees and attendings in practice, clinical performance is improved because of increased opportunities to review technical skills. This review could even occur just before performing a procedure. Chen and colleagues[34] demonstrated that residents performing a brief warm-up exercise on a laparoscopic simulator before a major or minor laparoscopic procedure had significantly improved intraoperative performance regardless of case difficulty. Incorporating frequent and thoughtful multidisciplinary simulation-based team training is an absolute necessity to streamline responses to rare and emergency events and to enhance communication. Lack of standardization and communication lapses are frequent contributors to preventable adverse outcomes. Finally, using in situ simulation to assess individual and team preparedness as well as the clinical environment will allow everyone to recognize and correct any deficiencies or modifiable systems issues proactively, before these gaps harm patients.

SUMMARY

Increasing focus on improving patient safety and outcomes in obstetrics and gynecology has stimulated interest in incorporating drills and simulation into medical training, continuing medical education, and team training. Drills and simulations are ideal tools because of their wide range of application with various learners and settings, providing a safe space to learn and maintain technical and communication skills, particularly for rare and complex clinical scenarios. The goal of drills and simulations in obstetrics and gynecology is to improve technical and communication skills, enhance teamwork, and build confidence. Ultimately, this will improve patient outcomes.

REFERENCES

1. Neuhauser D. Ernest Amory Codman MD. BMJ Qual Saf 2002;11:104–5.
2. AHRQ patient safety primer. Patient safety 101. Agency for Healthcare Research and Quality, Patient Safety Network; 2018. Available at: https://psnet.ahrq.gov/primers/primer/42/Patient-Safety-101. Accessed September 23, 2018.
3. Kohn LT, Corrigan JM, Donaldson MS. To err is human: building a safer health system. Washington, DC: National Academy Press; 1999.
4. Bates DW, Spell N, Cullen DJ, et al. Cost of adverse drug events in hospitalized patients. Adverse drug events prevention study group. JAMA 1997;277:307–11.
5. Philibert I, Friedmann P, Williams WT. for the members of the ACGME Work Group on resident duty hours. New requirements for resident duty hours. JAMA 2002; 288(9):1112–4.

6. DRILL definition in the Cambridge English Dictionary. 2018. Available at: Dictionary. cambridge.org; https://dictionary.cambridge.org/us/dictionary/english/drill. Accessed September 23, 2018.

7. American College of Obstetricians and Gynecologists Committee on Patient Safety and Quality Improvement. Committee Opinion No. 590. Preparing for clinical emergencies in obstetrics and gynecology. Obstet Gynecol 2014;123:722–5.

8. Flangan B, Nestel D, Joseph M. Making patient safety the focus: crisis resource management in the undergraduate curriculum. Med Educ 2004;38:56–66.

9. Al-Elq AH. Simulation-based medical teaching and learning. J Family Community Med 2010;17(1):35–40.

10. Rosen KR. The history of medical simulation. J Crit Care 2008;23(2):157–66.

11. Okuda Y, Bryson EO, DeMaria S Jr, et al. The utility of simulation in medical education: what is the evidence? Mt Sinai J Med 2009;76(4):330–43.

12. Ericsson KA. Deliberate practice and the acquisition and maintenance of expert performance in medicine and related domains. Acad Med 2004;79(10 Suppl): S70–81.

13. Li M, Liang Y. Wang Weiyi, acupuncture expert of the Song Dynasty. J Tradit Chin Med 2015;2(3):133–4.

14. Markoviç D, Markoviç-Živkoviç B. Development of anatomical models—chronology. Acta Med Median 2010;49:56–62.

15. Argani CH, Eichelberger M, Deering S, et al. The case for simulation as part of a comprehensive patient safety program. Am J Obstet Gynecol 2012;206(6):451–5.

16. American College of Obstetricians and Gynecologists Committee Committee on Patient Safety and Quality Improvement. ACOG Committee Opinion No. 447. Patient safety in obstetrics and gynecology. Obstet Gynecol 2009;114:1424–7.

17. Fanning RM, Gaba DM. The role of debriefing in simulation-based learning. Simul Healthc 2007;2(2):115–25.

18. Rudolph JW, Simon R, Dufresne R, et al. There's no such thing as "nonjudgmental" debriefing: a theory and method for debriefing with good judgment. Simul Healthc 2006;1:49–55.

19. Knowles M. What is andragogy?. In: The modern practice of adult education: from pedagogy to andragogy. San Francisco (CA): Jossey-Bass; 1980. p. 40–59.

20. Hopkins L, Hampton BS, Abbott JF, et al. To the point: medical education, technology, and the millennial learner. Am J Obstet Gynecol 2018;218(2):188–92.

21. Mahan J, Clinchot D. Why medical education is being (inexorably) re-imagined and re-designed. Curr Probl Pediatr Adolesc Health Care 2014;44:137–9.

22. Carpentio LJ. A lifetime commitment: mandatory continuing education. Nurs Times 1991;87:53–5.

23. Stross JK. Maintaining competency in advanced cardiac life support skills. JAMA 1983;24:3339–41.

24. O'Steen DS, Kee CC, Minick HP. The retention of advanced cardiac life support knowledge among registered nurses. J Nurs Staff Dev 1996;12:66–72.

25. Crofts JF, Ellis D, Draycott TJ, et al. Change in knowledge of midwives and obstetricians following obstetric emergency training: a randomised controlled trial of local hospital, simulation centre and teamwork training. BJOG 2007;114(12): 1534–41.

26. Ellis D, Crofts JF, Hunt LP, et al. Hospital, simulation center, and teamwork training for eclampsia management: a randomized controlled trial. Obstet Gynecol 2008; 111(3):723–31.

27. Crofts JF, Bartlett C, Ellis D, et al. Training for shoulder dystocia: a trial of simulation using low-fidelity and high-fidelity mannequins. Obstet Gynecol 2006;108(6): 1477–85.

28. Crofts JF, Bartlett C, Ellis D, et al. Patient-actor perception of care: a comparison of obstetric emergency training using manikins and patient-actors. Qual Saf Health Care 2008;17(1):20–4.

29. Crofts JF, Bartlett C, Ellis D, et al. Management of shoulder dystocia: skill retention 6 and 12 months after training. Obstet Gynecol 2007;110(5):1069–74.

30. Maslovitz S, Barkai G, Lessing JB, et al. Recurrent obstetric management mistakes identified by simulation. Obstet Gynecol 2007;109(6):1295–300.

31. Crofts JF, Lenguerrand E, Bentham GL, et al. Prevention of brachial plexus injury-12 years of shoulder dystocia training: an interrupted time-series study. BJOG 2016;123(1):111–8.

32. Siassakos D, Hasafa Z, Sibanda T, et al. Retrospective cohort study of diagnosis-delivery interval with umbilical cord prolapse: the effect of team training. BJOG 2009;116(8):1089–96.

33. Asoğlu MR, Achjian T, Akbilgiç O, et al. The impact of a simulation-based training lab on outcomes of hysterectomy. J Turk Ger Gynecol Assoc 2016;17(2):60–4.

34. Chen CC, Green IC, Colbert-Getz JM, et al. Warm-up on a simulator improves residents' performance in laparoscopic surgery: a randomized trial. Int Urogynecol J 2013;24(10):1615–22.

Creating Change at Scale

Quality Improvement Strategies used by the California Maternal Quality Care Collaborative

Cathie Markow, RN, MBA[a,b], Elliott K. Main, MD[a,c],*

KEYWORDS

- Quality improvement • Maternal mortality • Maternal morbidity
- Quality collaboratives • California maternal quality care collaborative

KEY POINTS

- Engagement of as many partners as possible in a quality improvement project leads to collective impact.
- Availability of a rapid-cycle low-burden data center is an important support for quality improvement activities.
- National safety bundles and tool kits provide guidance but need to be individualized to meet local resources.
- Working with other hospitals in a formal quality collaborative is an effective way to rapidly improve care.

Changing existing clinical practice has always been a challenging proposition. Medical leaders have lamented the fact that the average length of time required for national guidelines to be adopted into widespread practice is 17 years.[1] This sense of scientific advances being lost in translation underscores that medicine has powerful, homeostatic forces maintaining the status quo. In this discussion, the authors examine strategies that have shown the ability to markedly shorten the time for change and to be successful at scale. They examine 3 case studies of large-scale maternity quality

Disclosures: The authors have no commercial or financial conflicts of interest.
Funding Sources: Funding for the projects described in this report include California Department of Public Health, California Health Care Foundation, Merck for Mothers USA, and Centers for Disease Control and Prevention.
[a] California Maternal Quality Care Collaborative, Stanford University School of Medicine, Stanford Medical School Office Building, 1265 Welch Road, MS 5415, Stanford, CA 94305, USA;
[b] Division of Neonatal Medicine, Stanford University School of Medicine, Stanford, CA, USA;
[c] Department of Obstetrics and Gynecology, Stanford University School of Medicine, Stanford, CA, USA
* Corresponding author. California Maternal Quality Care Collaborative, Stanford Medical School Office Building, 1265 Welch Road, MS 5415, Stanford, CA 94305.
E-mail address: emain@stanford.edu

Obstet Gynecol Clin N Am 46 (2019) 317–328
https://doi.org/10.1016/j.ogc.2019.01.014
0889-8545/19/© 2019 Elsevier Inc. All rights reserved.

obgyn.theclinics.com

improvement (QI) projects undertaken by the California Maternal Quality Care Collaborative (CMQCC) that have shown success for problems that seemed difficult at the outset:

1. Early elective deliveries (EEDs)
2. Maternal mortality and severe maternal morbidity
3. Primary cesarean deliveries

All 3 of these problems developed gradually over a 20-year period, without a sudden increase, obscuring the origins and making the prior practice pattern seem distant. This observation of creeping statistics is reminiscent of the story about how to boil a frog without having it jump from the pot—gradually raise the temperature and the frog does not notice. Not surprisingly, creating a system for timely and transparent maternity data is 1 of the key principles for QI. The CMQCC model for achieving this progress has 3 additional key principles: multidisciplinary tool kits that provide best practices with implementation guidance; hands-on QI collaboratives and QI academies to support development of QI capacity; and establishment of a coalition of public and private partners all aligned to support the same project (**Fig. 1**).[2]

The first step, however, is to generate a shared vision for change—a compelling story or the proverbial burning platform—that creates an understanding that current practice is not sustainable. For greatest effectiveness, these calls to action involve a powerful combination of both data and stories. For EEDs, the authors used the high rates of neonatal ICU admissions prior to 37 weeks of gestation importantly paired with neonatologists describing local cases of severe respiratory morbidity among babies with repeat cesarean deliveries at 37 weeks of gestation. For maternal mortality and severe maternal morbidity, the authors used new California and US data showing a 50% to 70% rise of preventable maternal deaths combined with case vignettes of actual losses and near misses. For primary cesarean deliveries, the authors used the 50% rise in cesarean deliveries with no demonstrable improvement of infant outcomes and the astounding hospital variation of nulliparous term singleton vertex (NTSV) cesarean rates (ranging from 11% to 70% among California hospitals in 2014) combined with patient stories of placenta accreta and other major postcesarean complications.

The most powerful call for action has been maternal mortality. Over the past 2 decades, US maternal mortality rose significantly (to 15–23 per 100,000) whereas that in other high-resource countries fell.[3] Severe maternal morbidity as defined by the Centers for Disease Control and Prevention (CDC) has doubled in the same time period.[4] In 2006, noting a similar rise in California for maternal deaths and complications, the California Department of Public Health launched efforts to investigate maternal deaths, engage obstetric health providers, and expand regional coordination of care.[5] That year, CMQCC was formed as a public-private partnership, based at Stanford University, to lead maternal QI activities. The work began with the California Pregnancy-Associated Mortality Review. A multidisciplinary task force of experts conducted a detailed review of maternal deaths to determine cause of death, preventability, and, unusual for the time, clinical opportunities for improvement. The Mortality Review Committee assessment of preventability (defined as chance to alter the outcome) found 60% to 75% of leading causes of maternal death were preventable, as shown in **Fig. 2**. Hemorrhage and preeclampsia were identified as the causes with the highest preventability. They were also the leading causes of severe maternal morbidity and near misses.[6] They thus became the focus of the authors' first QI project to address maternal mortality. The utilization of California's maternal mortality data was an important driver for provider engagement.

TOOL KITS
Evidence-based
tool kits on leading
causes of
preventable
maternal morbidity
and mortality

MATERNAL
DATA CENTER
Near real-time
benchmarking
data to support
hospitals' quality
improvement

IMPLEMENTATION
Coaching on how
to implement best
practices and
sharing among
member hospitals

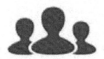

ENGAGEMENT
Engaging partners
around aligned
goals and
promoting
patient awareness

Fig. 1. The CMQCC 4 key principles for driving change.

The 4 principles for driving QI at scale are discussed as well as how they have been applied to each of the CMQCC major state-wide projects.

PRINCIPLE 1: ENGAGE AS MANY PARTNERS AS POSSIBLE: COLLECTIVE IMPACT IS POWERFUL

When the Maternal Mortality Review Committee examined the initial years of case reviews, CMQCC identified a pressing perinatal opportunity and undertook their first major initiative: elimination of EEDs.[7] The average gestational age at delivery for the entire United States had declined by more than 7 days between 1992 and 2002.[8] Much of the decline was due to scheduled inductions and cesarean deliveries prior to 39 weeks of gestation. Quickly it became clear that no 1 organization could successfully tackle this project but there was great opportunity for collective impact.

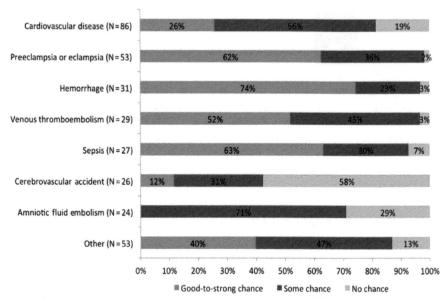

Fig. 2. Preventability of major causes of maternal mortality, California 2002 to 2007. (The California Pregnancy-Associated Mortality Review. Report from 2002-2007 Maternal Death Reviews. *Courtesy of* California Department of Public Health, Maternal, Child and Adolescent Health Division, Sacramento, CA. Available at: http:www.cdph.ca.gov/Programs/CFH/DMCAH/Pages/PAMR.aspx ©2017 California Department of Public Health.)

Many organizations have a greater effect than only 1 acting alone. CMQCC along with the March of Dimes and California Department of Public Health enlisted major professional organizations, the hospital association, health plans, and purchasers to join the collaborative. The multidisciplinary and multiorganization QI tool kit received letters of support from the American College of Obstetricians and Gynecologists (ACOG) and the Association of Women's Health, Obstetric and Neonatal Nurses (AWHONN), reinforcing its credibility for clinicians. Shortly afterward, The Joint Commission and the Centers for Medicare & Medicaid Services adopted national measures for EEDs, creating even more pressure on providers to change practice. Health plans began to pressure hospitals to eliminate these preventable cases of neonatal ICU admissions. The power of collaborative action leading to collective impact is shown in **Fig. 3**. No project goes unchallenged. Some physicians believed strongly that this project was an affront to provider autonomy. They eventually gave way to the multiple sources of leverage. **Fig. 4** shows CMQCC data illustrating the success at the population level after the project start in 2009. Eight years later, there were more than 200,000 cumulative fewer births between 35 and 38 or more weeks of gestation than would have occurred if the 2008 birth rates for each gestational age had continued.

The CMQCC projects to reduce maternal mortality and morbidity could not have succeeded without many organizations playing leading roles. The California Hospital Association and their affiliate, the Hospital Quality Institute, led efforts for hospital recruitment into the quality collaboratives. Major hospital systems embraced the projects and shared policies and educational materials broadly. Provider organizations enthusiastically supported the efforts and effectively used their

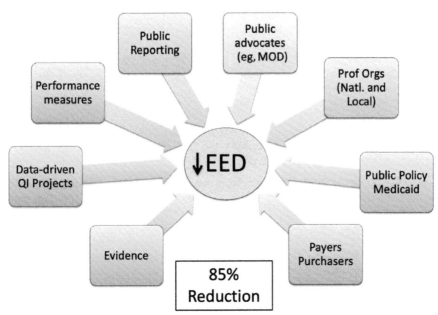

Fig. 3. Power of collaborative action leading to collective impact. This has been a key ingredient for the success of all of the CMQCC quality collaboratives. MOD, march of dimes; Prof Orgs (natal and Local), professional organizations (national and Local); EED, early elective delivery.

communication channels to promote the projects. More recently, health plans and Medi-Cal have provided incentives for adoption of hemorrhage and preeclampsia safety bundles.

Multipartner engagement and collective impact have also been central for the CMQCC current project: Supporting Vaginal Birth and Reducing Primary Cesareans.[9] The rate of cesareans deliveries increased by 50% from the late 1990's to 2012 in the United States and California. Given the 8% vaginal birth after cesarean rate, once a

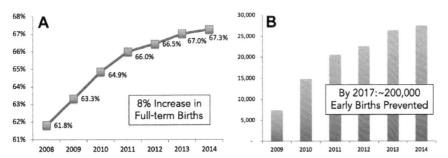

Fig. 4. Impact of the Eliminating Early Elective Deliveries Collaborative: the modest change in babies born after 39 weeks led to more than 200,000 fewer births between 35 weeks and 39 weeks from 2009 to 2017. (A) Percentage of full-term births in California (≥39 weeks' gestation). (B) Number of annual prevented births between greater than or equal to 35 weeks and less than 39 weeks. (Data from California Maternal Quality Care Collaborative (CMQCC). Maternal Data Center (MDC). Available at: https://www.cmqcc.org/maternal-data-center. Accessed November 15, 2018.)

woman has had a cesarean delivery, she has a 90% chance that all future deliveries will be by cesarean section, with the accompanying serious risks of placenta previa, placenta accreta, and uterine rupture. Even more than EEDs, decisions around cesarean birth have an impact on physician autonomy and, therefore, can be quite sensitive. This also was a setting for collective impact.

The power of engaging a broad set of partners cannot be understated nor should the effort required to do so. Having a strong value proposition along with a proved track record gets organizations to the table. Alignment on an aim with clear value for each of the partners is critical to engaging the partners and incorporating their leverage points in driving change. Similar to **Fig. 3** for EEDs, examples for the Supporting Vaginal Birth and Reducing Primary Cesareans include the following:

- CMQCC worked closely in an advisory role with Smart Care California, a public-private partnership of health plans and purchasers working to promote safe, affordable health care in California whose participants purchase or manage care for more than 16 million Californians—or 40% of the state's population. Smart Care participants used their purchasing power to bring attention to the issue of value-based purchasing specific to supporting vaginal birth.
- Health plans have initiated hospital performance incentives tied to the support of vaginal birth and achieving the Healthy People 2020 goal NTSV cesarean rate.
- Secretary of the California Health and Human Services Agency each year publicly recognized hospitals that have achieved the goal.
- Professional societies, such as ACOG and AWHONN, helped engage with their constituents through webinars and grand rounds.
- A partnership of the California Health Care Foundation, Consumer Reports, and CMQCC developed a set of publicly available patient education videos and content to align with the tool kit messaging that are available at www.mybirthmatters.org.

PRINCIPLE 2: MATERNAL DATA CENTER TO INFORM AND MANAGE QUALITY IMPROVEMENT

The CMQCC Maternal Data Center (MDC) provides rapid-cycle (as current as possible) hospital-level and provider-level data to support QI activities. The development of the MDC was funded by grants from the CDC and the California Health Care Foundation. Currently it is supported by fees from CMQCC member hospitals. In recent years, the MDC assisted state perinatal quality collaboratives in Washington and Oregon in addition to CMQCC. The MDC was designed to minimize hospital burden for data collection yet provide robust clinical information offering insights needed for QI and timely assessment of progress (or lack thereof). Hospital enthusiasm for the MDC is due to rapid-cycle data processing that is low burden/low cost (particularly for data collection/entry), flexible (because QI topics change), able to benchmark data in many ways (for example, to compare hospitals with similar levels of care or within similar geographies or compare providers within the same organization), and able to drill down to understand the underlying data and make necessary corrections. Just having the data center alone, however, is not enough. Having a knowledgeable support team to assist hospitals users is critical, especially with the significant turnover experienced by many labor and delivery units. CMQCC staff provided 1-on-1 support to hospitals as well as an ongoing series for Web trainings on the use of the data center.

To create a comprehensive maternal-infant data set, every month the MDC links birth certificate data with mother and infant hospital discharge diagnosis files

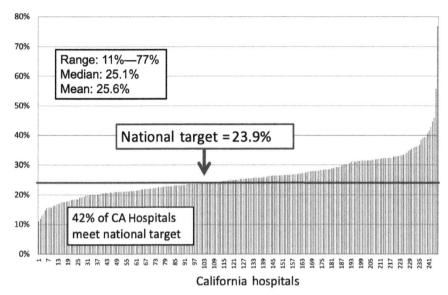

Fig. 5. Hospital variation of NTSV cesarean rates. All 248 California (CA) hospitals, 2015.

(minimizing burden by using already collected data) for all births at each member hospital. The system creates more than 50 maternal/infant performance measures and additional data quality tools. A Web-based user interface allows hospitals to access their data using data visualization strategies to promote multiple peer comparisons, benchmark in multiple ways, and track progress over time. A valuable approach within the data center is a focus on measure analysis, which allows facilities to analyze a measure understanding why it is elevated and then identify specific areas for QI. The Web portal also serves as the data entry site for all CMQCC QI collaboratives to collect, display, and compare both process and structure metrics.

The power of rapidly repurposing existing clinical information for QI is best illustrated by CMQCC's most recent project, Supporting Vaginal Birth and Reducing Primary Cesareans. The NTSV cesarean rate represents a reasonably standardized group of first births and have the highest risk for primary cesarean. It has been selected as the cesarean measure by National Quality Forum, The Joint Commission, Centers for Medicare & Medicaid Services, and Leapfrog Group, among others. The MDC can share and display California hospitals' NTSV cesarean rates. The variation is astonishing, with a range in 2015 from 11% to 77% (**Fig. 5**). The variation proved an important tool for engagement.

For cohorts of hospitals with NTSV cesarean rates above 23.9%, the MDC provided updates and benchmarking of current rates and safety and balancing measures. These included any unintended harm from the QI project—low Apgar scores or the neonatal composite (unexpected newborn complications), third-degree and fourth-degree lacerations, and operative vaginal deliveries. The MDC also provided an analysis of which subset of NTSV cesareans was driving the elevated rate (eg, spontaneous labor vs induced labor vs no labor) and within the labor categories, an analysis was provided for the cesarean indication.

There has been a decrease in the average low-risk, first-birth cesarean section rate from 25.5% (2015) to 24.5% (2017) for all California hospitals that deliver babies (n = 240) and to 23.6% (2Q2018) for all 208 hospitals with data in CMQCC MDC.

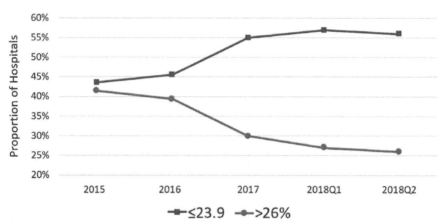

Fig. 6. The number of California hospitals with NTSV cesarean rates below 23.9% has increased significantly whereas the number of California hospitals with rates above 26% has fallen during the CMQCC Supporting Vaginal Birth and Reducing Primary Cesarean Collaborative that began in mid-2016.

The proportion of hospitals now achieving the goal has increased to 56% There has also been a proportionate reduction of hospitals with high NTSV cesarean rates that have now fallen below 27% (**Fig. 6**).

The MDC has served as the central tool for prior collaboratives examining hemorrhage and preeclampsia by providing immediate display and benchmarking of the main outcome measure, the CDC severe maternal morbidity rate, as well as measures of process and structure. As the sustainability phase of those projects has been moved to, the MDC provides continual surveillance of hospital and state rates of overall severe maternal morbidity as well as morbidity related to hemorrhage and hypertension. Recently the ability to follow rates of NTSV cesarean delivery and morbidity by race were added.

PRINCIPLE 3: TOOL KITS: GUIDANCE ON BEST PRACTICES

CMQCC Maternal Quality Improvement Toolkits aim to improve the health care response to leading causes of preventable death and severe complications among pregnant and postpartum women as well as reduce harm to infants and women from overuse of obstetric procedures. All tool kits include a compendium of best practice tools and articles, care guidelines in multiple formats, hospital-level implementation guide, and professional education slide set. The tool kits were developed in partnership with key experts from across California, representing the diverse professionals and institutions that care for pregnant and postpartum women.

Beginning in 2010, CMQCC with the California Department of Public Health (Maternal Child and Adolescent Health Division) and other partners published a series of tool kits to encourage maternity QI. The tool kits address EEDs (with the March of Dimes), obstetric hemorrhage (2 editions), hypertensive disorders, prevention of venous thromboembolism, cardiovascular disease in pregnancy, and supporting vaginal birth/reducing primary cesareans (with California Health Care Foundation and others).[10] Recent tool kits have been synchronized with the national patient safety bundles produced by the Council on Patient Safety in Women's Health Care.[11] The roles of quality tool kits and safety bundles are often confused. Bundles are essentially

Medications/ Procedures	Protocol/ Guideline	Safety Bundle	QI Toolkit

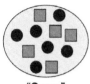

"Soup"	"Directions"	"Support Services"	"How-To Guide"

● **Meds:**
Oxy, Ergo, Prost, TXA, Blood

■ **Procs:**
D&C, Balloon, B-Lynch, IR, NASG, Hyst

A start, but not nearly enough to lead change by itself

1. **Make it easy**
   Hem Cart, Order sets, Posters
2. **Communications**
   Risk Assess, QBL, Situation Awareness
3. **Teamwork**
   Drills, Broad Engage.
4. **System Learning**
   Debriefs, Case Reviews

Implementation resources, advice, examples

Collaborative Sharing

Fig. 7. Making sense of QI tools: using obstetric hemorrhage to illustrate the differences between protocols/guidelines, safety bundles, and QI tool kits. OXY, oxytocin; Ergo, ergotamine; Prost, prostaglandins; TXA, tranexamic acid; D&C, dilation and curettage; B-Lynch, B-Lynch suture; IR, interventional radiology; NASG, non-pneumatic anti-shock garment; Hyst, hysterectomy.

a structured list of best practices that should be addressed for all birthing facilities. Tool kits provide the necessary details, rationale, and implementation materials, such as sample policies and protocols. **Fig. 7** provides a comparison of protocols, bundles, and tool kits that will provide more clarification using obstetric hemorrhage as an example.

As another example, the *Toolkit to Support Vaginal Birth and Reduce Primary Cesareans* is a comprehensive, evidence-based guide designed to educate and motivate maternity clinicians in the implementation of best practices for supporting vaginal birth.[12] The focus is on cesarean births among low-risk, first-time mothers, the largest contributor to the recent rise in cesarean rates, and accounts for the greatest variation in cesarean rates between hospitals.

The tool kit contains key strategies and resources to

- Improve the culture of care, awareness, and education for cesarean reduction
- Support intended vaginal birth
- Manage labor abnormalities and safely reduce cesarean births
- Use data to drive reduction in cesareans

PRINCIPLE 4: IMPLEMENTATION GUIDANCE FOR SUCCESSFUL ENGAGEMENT AND IMPROVEMENT

The success of the hospitals in reducing their severe maternal morbidity or their first birth cesarean rate is dependent on the engagement and dedication of their clinical staff. Not all labor and delivery units, however, have the QI experience or leadership skills needed to drive the work. For the authors' large collaboratives (>30 hospitals at 1 time), CMQCC organizes 8 to 10 hospitals into groups and assigns an experienced physician and nurse coach/mentor team to work with them over a period of 18 months to implement the strategies found in the tool kit and to facilitate the sharing of promising ideas formulated by the participating hospitals.[13] CMQCC follows a modified Institute for Healthcare Improvement Breakthrough Series model.[14] The process begins with an in-person kickoff meeting where key concepts are introduced, and group members have an opportunity to meet each other. The groups then meet via monthly webinars facilitated by the mentors and CMQCC clinical staff, to share learnings, challenges, and achievements with each other. The mentors are expected to make at least 1 site visit to each of the hospitals, often participating in grand rounds as a means of personally engaging the clinical staff. At the end of the 18 months, a second in-person meeting is held to celebrate and share the achievements of each of the participating hospitals.

The formal collaborative is supported by an active LISTSERV, where participating hospitals can share ideas, questions, and help each other. In addition, regular educational webinars are presented on topics, such as new research, and labor support techniques. The CMQCC team includes experienced nurse educators, physicians, nursing directors, and midwives who coordinate the project as a whole. Specifically, they work with all the mentor groups, sharing information between groups and providing 1-on-1 assistance to hospitals as needed.

While working with more than 200 hospitals on QI collaboratives, the authors have observed that many facilities, especially their maternity physician and nursing leaders, did not have much, if any experience, with QI techniques and practices. Furthermore, it became apparent that change management and specific techniques do not come naturally for many professionals. The authors were able to teach some approaches during each collaborative. Recently the authors initiated a QI academy to teach QI techniques to multidisciplinary leadership teams from 10 to 12 hospitals at a time. The curriculum focuses on techniques, such as driver diagrams, run charts, data analysis, and models for leading change. The academy uses examples and principles from John Kotter's *8-step Process for Leading Change*,[15] Joseph Grenny and colleagues' *Influencer: the new science of leading change*,[16] and Chip Heath and Dan Heath's *Switch: How to Change Things when Change is Hard*.[17] The course is structured as a learning collaborative, with every team using these techniques to promote changes on their unit.

Not surprisingly, sustainability has become an issue for the authors' facilities. Staff turnover, of both nurses and physicians, necessitates continual education and surveillance to prevent backsliding on gains made during the formal collaboratives. To address this very real issue, the authors are using variety of tools. The data center automatically tracks a set of measures using administrative data. These measure then serve as alarms when there is a change for the worse. Partners continue to encourage and reward transparency and public attention to their outcome measures. The authors are developing a set of brief educational updates and Web-based materials to keep the key principles current with new hires. Nationally, the Alliance for Innovation on Maternal Health (AIM) is also developing web-modules and other useful materials with its set of national partners that will be available for all hospitals and be particularly valuable to sustain gains.[18]

Funding for CMQCC began with contracts from the California Department of Public Health using Title V Maternal and Child Health Services Block Grant Program funds. Over time, CDC and private foundation grants were added to develop the MDC and develop new programs. In its tenth year, CMQCC membership benefits (eg, MDC, QI projects, and educational activities) have proved of value to hospitals that pay modest membership fees. Given the demonstrated improvements in population health illustrated in this report, several health plans are now providing financial incentives for hospitals to join CMQCC. The CMQCC members now include hospitals that account for more than 96% of California births. Currently the authors' funding model is a combination of grants and member hospital fees. Thea authors expect that new programs will be supported by grants whereas member fees help support core costs, such as staff and infrastructure.

SUMMARY

There is no 1 tactic that drives a successful QI project. It takes data to demonstrate a need, to provide guidance on where to focus resources, and to show progress. Partnerships are critical. True collective impact can be achieved with a wide variety of stakeholders who share the vision and goals and who can leverage their relationships in support of those goals. A common scientific and educational base in the form of QI tool kits and, more recently, tool kits combined with national safety bundles provides common language and approaches for implementation. Finally, implementation training and education to develop expertise and build QI capacity is a long-term endeavor, allowing QI to flourish. Ultimately it is the physicians, nurse leaders, and their peers who do the hard work of changing clinical practice, improving quality of care, and reducing maternal mortality and morbidity.

REFERENCES

1. Lenfant C. Clinical research to clinical practice—lost in translation? N Engl J Med 2003;349:868–74.
2. Main EK, Markow C, Gould J. Addressing maternal mortality and morbidity in California through public-private partnerships. Health Aff 2018;37:1484–93.
3. Creanga AA, Syverson C, Seed K, et al. Pregnancy-related mortality in the United States,2011-2013. Obstet Gynecol 2017;130:366–73.
4. Centers for Disease Control. Severe maternal mortality in the United States. Atlanta (GA): Centers for Disease Control; 2017. Available at: www.cdc.gov/reproductivehealth/maternalinfanthealth/severematernalmorbidity.html. Accessed November 15, 2018.
5. California Department of Public Health. Center for family health, maternal, Child and Adolescent Health Division. Maternal mortality rate: California and the United States, 1999-2013 2015. Available at: https://www.cmqcc.org/research/maternal-mortality-review-ca-pamr/ca-pamr-process-and-publications. Accessed November 15, 2018.
6. Main EK, McCain CL, Morton CH, et al. Pregnancy related mortality in California: causes, characteristics, and improvement opportunities. Obstet Gynecol 2015; 125(4):938–47.
7. Main E, Oshiro B, Chagolla B, et al. Elimination of non–medically indicated (elective) deliveries before 39 weeks gestational age: a California toolkit to transform maternity care. Stanford (CA): California Maternal Quality Care Collaborative; 2011 (Developed with the California Department of Public Health). Available at: https://www.cmqcc.org/resources-tool-kits/toolkits/early-elective-deliveries-toolkit. Accessed November 15, 2018.
8. Davidoff MJ, Dias T, Damus K, et al. Changes in the gestational age distribution among U.S. singleton births: impact on rates of late preterm birth, 1992 to 2002. Semin Perinatol 2006;30:8–15.
9. Smith H, Peterson N, Lagrew D, et al. California Maternal Quality Care Collaborative (CMQCC). Toolkit to support vaginal birth and reduce primary cesareans: a

quality improvement toolkit. Available at: https://www.cmqcc.org/VBirthToolkit. Accessed November 15, 2018.

10. CMQCC: maternal quality improvement toolkits. Available at: https://www.cmqcc. org/resources-tool-kits/toolkits. Accessed November 15, 2018

11. Council on Patient Safety in Women's Health Care. Patient safety bundles. Washington, DC. Available at: https://safehealthcareforeverywoman.org/patient-safety-bundles/. Accessed November 15, 2018.

12. CMQCC. Toolkit to support vaginal birth and reduce primary cesareans. Available at: https://www.cmqcc.org/VBirthToolkit. Accessed November 15, 2018.

13. Main EK, Dhurjati R, Cape V, et al. Improving maternal safety at scale with the mentor model of collaborative improvement. Jt Comm J Qual Patient Saf 2018; 44(5):250–9.

14. Institute for Healthcare Improvement. The Breakthrough Series: IHI's collaborative model for achieving breakthrough improvement. Boston: IHI; 2003 (registration required) Available at: http://www.ihi.org/knowledge/Pages/IHIWhitePapers/ TheBreakthroughSeriesIHIsCollaborativeModelforAchievingBreakthroughImprove ment.aspx. Accessed November 15, 2018.

15. Kotter J. 8-step process for leading change. Available at: https://www.kotterinc. com/8-steps-process-for-leading-change/. Accessed November 15, 2018.

16. Grenny J, Patterson K, Maxfield D, et al. Influencer: the new science of leading change. 2nd edition. New York: McGraw-Hill; 2013.

17. Heath C, Heath D. Switch: how to change when change is hard. New York: Broadway Books; 2010.

18. Alliance for Innovation on Maternal Health Program (AIM). Available at: https:// safehealthcareforeverywoman.org/aim-program/. Accessed November 15, 2018.

Obstetric Anesthesia
Leading the Way in Patient Safety

David J. Birnbach, MD, MPH[a],*, Brian T. Bateman, MD, MSc[b]

KEYWORDS

- Patient safety • Obstetric anesthesia • Neuraxial blockade • Epidural analgesia

KEY POINTS

- The field of anesthesiology has been a leader in patient safety.
- Obstetric anesthesia has a long history of advancing patient safety and continues to lead in this area.
- Team training is a major advance in patient safety for the labor and delivery suite.

Although anesthesiologists comprise only approximately 5% of physicians practicing in the United States, the specialty is acknowledged as a leader in patient safety.[1] The practice of anesthesia is far safer today than it was just a few decades ago. Contemporary practice bears little resemblance to that of the 1950s and 1960s. Studies in the in 1970s and 1980s shed light on anesthesia-related issues that were associated with preventable patient harm, and solutions. Technological advances, including the advent of pulse oximetry, capnography, airway management aids, such as laryngeal mask airway and videolaryngoscopy, along with improvements in drugs markedly reduced the risk associated with general anesthesia.[2,3] Anesthesiologists embraced this new safer future and dramatically changed the way that they practiced. Leading this movement, the Anesthesia Patient Safety Foundation, which was created in 1985, articulated the vision that "no patient shall be harmed by anesthesia." Its founders coined the term "patient safety" in its modern public usage.[4]

The subspecialty of obstetric anesthesiology has embraced patient safety research leading to a reduction in obstetric anesthesia-related morbidity and mortality.[5,6] This tradition has deep roots. As far back as 1847, Sir James Young Simpson introduced general anesthesia for labor (ether) while questioning the unintended consequences of anesthesia including fetal well-being.[7] A century later, Virginia Apgar while working as

Disclosure Statement: No conflicts.
[a] University of Miami–Jackson Memorial Hospital Center for Patient Safety, University of Miami Miller School of Medicine, 1611 Northwest 12th Avenue, C-300, Miami, FL 33136, USA;
[b] Division of Obstetric Anesthesia, Department of Anesthesiology, Brigham and Women's Hospital, Harvard Medical School, 75 Francis Street, Boston, MA 02115, USA
* Corresponding author.
E-mail address: dbirnbach@miami.edu

an obstetric anesthesiologist in the 1950s called into question the widespread practice of "twilight sleep" (scopolamine plus morphine) for labor analgesia. She was an early pioneer of neuraxial blockade for labor (caudal) as a safer alternative to twilight sleep. She developed the Apgar score, and then used the data to illuminate the benefits of neuraxial blockade as compared with parenteral medications. Epidural analgesia, reintroduced in the 1970s, presented a further major step in producing a safer technique to provide labor analgesia. Many other examples of anesthesiology, in general and obstetric anesthesia specifically, that lead the way in patient safety abound.

Although there are innumerable individual improvements that have produced the safe practice that is provided by obstetric anesthesiologists today, this review highlight the following innovations:

1. Safer and more effective labor analgesia.
2. Safer treatments for hypotension associated with neuraxial blockade.
3. Advances in spinal and epidural techniques for operative deliveries.
4. Lower incidence of postdural puncture headache through improved technology.
5. Safer parental agents for labor analgesia.
6. Improved safety of general anesthesia in obstetrics.
7. Improved education and the use of simulation including team training.
8. Reductions in operating room (OR)-related infections.

SAFER AND MORE EFFECTIVE LABOR ANALGESIA

In the 1970s and 1980s neuraxial analgesia for labor was typically provided with a labor epidural, which was dosed every few hours when the desired anesthetic effect wore off. The local anesthetic of choice was often concentrated enough to cause a solid sensory block, but also caused a significant degree of motor blockade and marked hypotension. The methods for administering labor analgesia have changed numerous times in the ensuing 40 years. Now continuous infusions of dilute local anesthetics with the addition of a low concentration of opioid are used to produce stable levels of analgesia while reducing the need for bolus administration of medications for breakthrough pain.[8] Problems with dense motor block are less common and marked hypotension is rarely seen. Patient-controlled administration options are commonly used in addition to continuous infusions. Analgesia provided with this approach is superior while at the same time associated with lower incidence of motor block and a lower total local anesthetic dose consumption.[9]

What does this have to do with leading the way in patient safety? First, anesthesiologists had the self-awareness that old approaches to managing epidurals were not perfect and needed to be improved. Second, they listened to the voices of key stakeholders including obstetricians, labor nurses, and parturients regarding characteristics of an ideal analgesic block. Third, with better and safer labor analgesia using neuraxial catheter techniques, the epidural rate for laboring women increased. Those epidural catheters can also be used to provide an anesthetic for cesarean delivery. The increased use of neuraxial blocks and subsequent decreased use of general anesthesia for cesarean delivery, improved safety.

Obstetric anesthesiologists also demonstrated improved obstetric outcomes by use of epidural analgesia. For example, a large randomized control trial by Wong and coworkers[10] debunked the notion that neuraxial analgesia initiated in early labor increased the rate of cesarean delivery. They found that the rate of cesarean delivery was comparable in those randomized to early versus late initiation of neuraxial analgesia. Additionally, labor was shorter and analgesia better in the early group. More recently, a randomized controlled trial by Shen and colleagues[11] demonstrated that maintaining epidural analgesia during the second stage of labor using a dilute, motor-sparing local anesthetic infusion did not increase the length of the second stage or the rate of successful vaginal delivery.

SAFER TREATMENTS FOR HYPOTENSION ASSOCIATED WITH NEURAXIAL BLOCKADE

Hypotension is much less commonly associated with the provision of neuraxial analgesia for labor as compared with spinal anesthesia for cesarean delivery. Treatment, however, is still necessary especially when dense neuraxial blocks to provide anesthesia for cesarean deliveries reach higher dermatomal levels and are associated with sympathetic blockade. Beginning in the 1970s, ephedrine became the predominantly used pressor agent to treat neuraxial technique-related hypotension. This preference for ephedrine instead of phenylephrine was because of evidence-based data evaluating uterine blood flow in pregnant ewes.[12] For more than 20 years, ephedrine was often the only choice of drug to treat hypotension in the parturient. The pendulum swung in the 1990s when newer, relevant human evidence (eg, Doppler evaluations of uterine blood flow) found that phenylephrine was safe and effective, and ephedrine had potential negative impacts on the fetus.[13] Anesthesiologists sought to reexamine dogma and use newer technology to help find safer treatment options.

ADVANCES IN SPINAL AND EPIDURAL TECHNIQUES FOR OPERATIVE DELIVERIES

The 1980s saw a dramatic increase in the use of neuraxial blockade for cesarean delivery. At first, the use of neuraxial anesthesia was not nearly as safe as it is today. During this period, bupivacaine was introduced into obstetric practice with the promise of better sensory blockade and less motor block. Unfortunately, several cases of maternal mortality occurred when large bolus doses of 0.75% epidural bupivacaine administered through an unrecognized intravascular catheter caused a cardiac arrest.[14] Since that time, processes have been put into place, along with development of new drugs, to dramatically reduce this risk. These include removal of 0.75% epidural bupivacaine from use in obstetric anesthesia, use of test doses (to identify catheters inadvertently threaded into blood vessels or the intrathecal space), incremental bolus administration, and the availability of an intralipid antidote to local anesthetic toxicity.[15] This is another example on the part of the obstetric anesthesia community of identifying a safety issue, understanding the problem, and fixing it.

Similarly, spinal anesthesia techniques have gone through significant changes to increase its safety. Not only have safer agents (eg, 0.75% hyperbaric bupivacaine for subarachnoid block) gained in popularity, but less safe agents with greater potential risks, such as tetracaine with its associated risk of high spinals, and hyperbaric lidocaine plus epinephrine with its risk of neurotoxicity, are no longer regularly used.

DECREASING THE INCIDENCE OF POSTDURAL PUNCTURE HEADACHE THROUGH IMPROVED TECHNOLOGY

The anesthesia community has also been at the forefront of developing and using spinal needles that are associated with dramatically lower incidences of postdural puncture headache. Postdural puncture headaches, which have been called "the worst common complication in obstetric anesthesia,"[16] have almost disappeared following spinal anesthesia because of the use of these new spinal needles. These needles, commonly termed "pencil point," spread rather than cut dural fibers.[17] In addition, a large part of patient safety involves disseminating the message so that others can benefit. Not only have these needles become the default needles for use in obstetric anesthesia, but the anesthesia community has also shared their knowledge with other specialties who also perform lumbar puncture, such as neurologists.[18]

SAFER PARENTAL AGENTS FOR LABOR ANALGESIA

Although the safest and most effective method for providing labor pain relief is a neuraxial block,[19] not every parturient can receive one. This is related to staffing issues,[20] patient refusal, or contraindications to these blocks (eg, the parturient with a coagulopathy). If analgesia is requested in such a patient, the current choices for parenteral medications are far superior compared with those that were offered in the past. Whereas pethidine (Demerol) given intramuscularly was the gold standard for many years and is still commonly used in some countries,[21] fentanyl and remifentanil likely offer safer and more effective alternatives. The use of these medications still requires close patient monitoring.

There is still some controversy regarding the risks and benefits of remifentanil. A recent survey reported that approximately one-third of responding obstetric units had used remifentanil patient-controlled intravenous analgesia (PCIA) in the past 12 months.[22] An accompanying editorial suggested that safety remained an issue and recommended that "although remifentanil PCIA might be the best nonneuraxial strategy in terms of analgesic quality, patient safety hazards are significant, and a careful risk–benefit analysis does not support its routine use."[23] That said, a recent high-profile study demonstrated that inadequate pain relief (measured by the requirement for epidural pain relief) was dramatically lower in women who received remifentanil PCIA compared with intramuscular pethidine. An increased proportion of low maternal oxygen saturation and additional requirement for oxygen supplementation was observed with remifentanil; however, it did not result in adverse maternal or neonatal sequelae.[24] Regardless of the agent chosen, these newer and stronger opioids should be used only by those with adequate training and ability to perform reversal and resuscitation.

IMPROVED SAFETY OF GENERAL ANESTHESIA IN OBSTETRICS

General anesthesia has long been feared as a leading cause of maternal mortality. Ongoing morbidity and mortality studies identify cases of failed intubation and aspiration associated with general anesthesia.[25] General anesthesia increases the risk for death at the time of cesarean delivery. Before the availability of modern tools that increase the safety of airway management, general anesthesia was associated with 16.7 times the mortality of neuraxial anesthesia.[6] These tools include better monitoring (pulse oximetry and capnography), better laryngoscopes (eg, videolaryngoscopy), airway adjuncts (laryngeal mask airways and combitubes), and better training (eg, simulation-based drills).[26] In addition, the American Society of Anesthesiologists developed and disseminated an algorithm to facilitate responding to a difficult intubation. This stepwise, standardized approach has undoubtedly reduced the incidence of failed intubation leading to maternal death.[27] Team training has also reduced morbidity and mortality.[28]

Aspiration pneumonitis was a major cause of anesthesia-related maternal mortality in the 1940s and 1950s.[29] Several practice changes embraced by the anesthesia community along with better technology have resulted in a dramatic reduction of aspiration. These included the widespread use of neuraxial anesthesia, oral intake restrictions in labor, preanesthetic antacid administration, rapid sequence induction of general anesthesia, improvement in anesthesia training, and improvements in advanced airway devices.[5]

IMPROVED EDUCATION AND THE USE OF SIMULATION INCLUDING TEAM TRAINING

Simulation-based education has improved the safety of obstetric anesthesia practice.[30] The use of general anesthetics for cesarean delivery has significantly decreased.[31] As a result, there is less opportunity for tomorrow's practitioners to learn how to manage difficult airways and failed intubations. Simulation-based training is perhaps the only way to prepare them to deal with these rare, life-threatening emergencies.[26] The effectiveness of this training is demonstrated by Goodwin and French,[32] who showed significant improvement from baseline in management of failed intubations after participation in simulated intubation drills. Significant improvement has also been reported following simulation-based education when evaluating the performance of cardiopulmonary resuscitation in the parturient. Simulation-based education also improves the accuracy of estimating intraoperative blood loss during cesarean delivery. Toledo and colleagues[33,34] found that during simulated massive maternal hemorrhage, clinicians underestimated maternal blood loss by as much as 59%. The underestimates were even greater as the actual blood loss increased. Following lectures on blood loss, and simulation-based training, the average underestimation decreased to only 4%.

In the past, simulation has been principally used in obstetric anesthesia to teach individual skills.[26] Now, there is an increased recognition that team training is essential for a high functioning labor and delivery unit. Simulation offers the perfect opportunity to practice the skills needed to function as a team. According to Pratt,[26] "the teamwork training is generally embedded into the simulation of an emergent clinical event, thus allowing the learners to practice the clinical and teamwork skills." Gum and colleagues[35] reported that simulation-based team training improved teamwork skills, including leadership and collaboration. Simulation-based education is used for resident teaching and their assessment. Scavone and colleagues[36] reported an objective scoring system for measurement of resident performance during simulations.

There is also a growing movement toward the effective use of crisis checklists, emergency manuals, and other cognitive aids in the OR.[37] These cognitive aids have been in use by high-reliability and high-performing industries for many years but only recently used in ORs. There is little evidence that their use has been routinely implemented on labor and delivery suites. Unfortunately, evidence suggests that failure to adhere to best practices during emergencies is common.[38,39] Anesthesiologists can play a key role in not only embracing checklists, but also in championing their use on labor and delivery suites. An example is keeping local anesthesia systemic toxicity checklists available in all areas where local anesthetics are used similar to malignant hyperthermia checklists being available wherever general anesthesia is administered.[40]

REDUCTION OF OPERATING ROOM–RELATED INFECTIONS

Health care–associated infection affects approximately 10% of patients admitted to acute care facilities, accounting for approximately 500,000 infections annually.[41] Labor and delivery suites and ORs are no exception. There are numerous studies that show that ORs are not sterile environments and that some postoperative infections are traced to contamination in the OR.[42] Anesthesiologists' inadequate hand hygiene has been shown to play a role in the transmission of infection.[43] Studies have now focused on methods to reduce the risk of OR contamination. One of those steps is the sheathing of the laryngoscope after intubation, so as to decrease the risk of contamination of the OR by the contaminated laryngoscope.[43] Comprehensive infection control programs also include use of personalized alcohol dispenser for more frequent hand hygiene in the OR, improved environmental cleaning, vascular care bundles, and greater infection surveillance. This is another area where anesthesiologists, along with other specialties, are working collaboratively to resolve this patient safety issue.[44]

FUTURE DIRECTIONS

The practice of obstetric anesthesia is now remarkably safe in the United States and other high-income countries. Anesthesia-related mortality is now exceedingly rare. Unfortunately, data suggest that the gains in safety that have occurred over the past half century in high-income countries have not been realized in low- and middle-income countries. A recent meta-analysis by Sobhy and colleagues[45] estimated that in these countries the risk of death from anesthesia is 1.2 per 1000. Anesthesia contributed to 3.5% of all direct maternal deaths and 13.8% of deaths after cesarean delivery. Failed tracheal intubation, pulmonary aspiration, and high spinal block accounted for a large fraction of these deaths. All of these complications could be significantly reduced by safety improvements in practice.[45]

There is also important work still to be done here in the United States. Although obstetric anesthesia is now remarkably safe, evidence suggests that labor floors are still not always meeting patient safety goals.[46,47] To achieve these goals collaboration between all members of the labor and delivery team, including anesthesiologists, obstetricians, and nurses, is necessary. Recently, Abir and Mhyre[48] reviewed the increasing maternal mortality rates in the United States and provided an overview of strategies to create an institutional culture of safety and equity. These included multidisciplinary team training, simulation, and shared decision making. Anesthesiologists play a key role working as members of this team. This is especially true in cases of severe preeclampsia, eclampsia, hemorrhage, or critically ill patients where anesthesiologist exercise their role as "peridelivery physicians."[49–52]

Anesthesiologists have been leaders in patient safety. This leadership has had a major impact on labor and delivery suites across the country. However, the journey is still in its infancy and much work remains to be done to fulfill the promise that "no patient shall be harmed by anesthesia." Safety is a never-ending process.[53]

REFERENCES

1. Gaba DM. Anaesthesiology as a model for patient safety in health care. BMJ 2000;320(7237):785–8.
2. Cooper JB, Newbower RS, Kitz RJ. An analysis of major errors and equipment failures in anesthesia management: considerations for prevention and detection. Anesthesiology 1984;60(1):34–42.
3. Derrington MC, Smith G. A review of studies of anaesthetic risk, morbidity and mortality. Br J Anaesth 1987;59(7):815–33.
4. Eichhorn JH. The Anesthesia Patient Safety Foundation at 25: a pioneering success in safety, 25th anniversary provokes reflection, anticipation. Anesth Analg 2012;114(4):791–800.
5. Lim G, Facco FL, Nathan N, et al. A review of the impact of obstetric anesthesia on maternal and neonatal outcomes. Anesthesiology 2018;129(1):192–215.
6. Hawkins JL, Chang J, Palmer SK, et al. Anesthesia-related maternal mortality in the United States: 1979-2002. Obstet Gynecol 2011;117(1):69–74.

7. Caton D. John Snow's practice of obstetric anesthesia. Anesthesiology 2000; 92(1):247–52.
8. Ginosar Y, Davidson EM, Firman N, et al. A randomized controlled trial using patient-controlled epidural analgesia with 0.25% versus 0.0625% bupivacaine in nulliparous labor: effect on analgesia requirement and maternal satisfaction. Int J Obstet Anesth 2010;19(2):171–8.
9. Practice guidelines for obstetric anesthesia: an updated report by the American Society of Anesthesiologists Task Force on Obstetric Anesthesia and the Society for Obstetric Anesthesia and Perinatology. Anesthesiology 2016;124(2):270–300.
10. Wong CA, Scavone BM, Peaceman AM, et al. The risk of cesarean delivery with neuraxial analgesia given early versus late in labor. N Engl J Med 2005;352(7): 655–65.
11. Shen X, Li Y, Xu S, et al. Epidural analgesia during the second stage of labor: a randomized controlled trial. Obstet Gynecol 2017;130(5):1097–103.
12. Ralston DH, Shnider SM, DeLorimier AA. Effects of equipotent ephedrine, meta-raminol, mephentermine, and methoxamine on uterine blood flow in the pregnant ewe. Anesthesiology 1974;40(4):354–70.
13. Ngan Kee WD, Lee A, Khaw KS, et al. A randomized double-blinded comparison of phenylephrine and ephedrine infusion combinations to maintain blood pressure during spinal anesthesia for cesarean delivery: the effects on fetal acid-base status and hemodynamic control. Anesth Analg 2008;107(4):1295–302.
14. Albright GA. Cardiac arrest following regional anesthesia with etidocaine or bupivacaine. Anesthesiology 1979;51(4):285–7.
15. Park WK, Kim HS, Kim SH, et al. Intralipid restoration of myocardial contractions following bupivacaine-induced asystole: concentration- and time-dependence in vitro. Anesth Analg 2017;125(1):91–100.
16. Sachs A, Smiley R. Post-dural puncture headache: the worst common complication in obstetric anesthesia. Semin Perinatol 2014;38(6):386–94.
17. Vallejo MC, Mandell GL, Sabo DP, et al. Postdural puncture headache: a randomized comparison of five spinal needles in obstetric patients. Anesth Analg 2000; 91(4):916–20.
18. Birnbach DJ, Kuroda MM, Sternman D, et al. Use of atraumatic spinal needles among neurologists in the United States. Headache 2001;41(4):385–90.
19. ACOG Committee Opinion #295: pain relief during labor. Obstet Gynecol 2004; 104(1):213.
20. Birnbach DJ, Bucklin BA, Dexter F. Impact of anesthesiologists on the incidence of vaginal birth after cesarean in the United States: role of anesthesia availability, productivity, guidelines, and patient safety. Semin Perinatol 2010;34(5):318–24.
21. Kranke P, Weibel S. Pain relief during labour: challenging the use of intramuscular pethidine. Lancet 2018;392(10148):617–9.
22. Aaronson J, Abramovitz S, Smiley R, et al. A survey of intravenous remifentanil use for labor analgesia at academic medical centers in the United States. Anesth Analg 2017;124(4):1208–10.
23. Van de Velde M. Remifentanil patient-controlled intravenous analgesia for labor pain relief: is it really an option to consider? Anesth Analg 2017;124(4):1029–31.
24. Wilson MJA, MacArthur C, Hewitt CA, et al. Intravenous remifentanil patient-controlled analgesia versus intramuscular pethidine for pain relief in labour (RESPITE): an open-label, multicentre, randomised controlled trial. Lancet 2018;392(10148):662–72.

25. Neuhaus S, Neuhaus C, Fluhr H, et al. "Why mothers die." Learning from the analysis of anaesthesia-related maternal deaths (1985-2013). Anaesthesist 2016; 65(4):281–94 [in German].

26. Pratt SD. Focused review: simulation in obstetric anesthesia. Anesth Analg 2012; 114(1):186–90.

27. Hagberg CA, Gabel JC, Connis RT. Difficult Airway Society 2015 guidelines for the management of unanticipated difficult intubation in adults: not just another algorithm. Br J Anaesth 2015;115(6):812–4.

28. Morgan PJ, Pittini R, Regehr G, et al. Evaluating teamwork in a simulated obstetric environment. Anesthesiology 2007;106(5):907–15.

29. Mendelson CL. The aspiration of stomach contents into the lungs during obstetric anesthesia. Am J Obstet Gynecol 1946;52:191–205.

30. Birnbach DJ, Salas E. Can medical simulation and team training reduce errors in labor and delivery? Anesthesiol Clin 2008;26(1):159–68, viii.

31. Tsen LC, Pitner R, Camann WR. General anesthesia for cesarean section at a tertiary care hospital 1990-1995: indications and implications. Int J Obstet Anesth 1998;7(3):147–52.

32. Goodwin MW, French GW. Simulation as a training and assessment tool in the management of failed intubation in obstetrics. Int J Obstet Anesth 2001;10(4): 273–7.

33. Toledo P, McCarthy RJ, Hewlett BJ, et al. The accuracy of blood loss estimation after simulated vaginal delivery. Anesth Analg 2007;105(6):1736–40, table of contents.

34. Toledo P, McCarthy RJ, Burke CA, et al. The effect of live and web-based education on the accuracy of blood-loss estimation in simulated obstetric scenarios. Am J Obstet Gynecol 2010;202(4):400.e1-5.

35. Gum L, Greenhill J, Dix K. Clinical simulation in maternity (CSiM): interprofessional learning through simulation team training. Qual Saf Health Care 2010; 19(5):e19.

36. Scavone BM, Sproviero MT, McCarthy RJ, et al. Development of an objective scoring system for measurement of resident performance on the human patient simulator. Anesthesiology 2006;105(2):260–6.

37. Hepner DL, Arriaga AF, Cooper JB, et al. Operating room crisis checklists and emergency manuals. Anesthesiology 2017;127(2):384–92.

38. Smith KK, Gilcreast D, Pierce K. Evaluation of staff's retention of ACLS and BLS skills. Resuscitation 2008;78(1):59–65.

39. McEvoy MD, Field LC, Moore HE, et al. The effect of adherence to ACLS protocols on survival of event in the setting of in-hospital cardiac arrest. Resuscitation 2014;85(1):82–7.

40. Neal JM, Bernards CM, Butterworth JF 4th, et al. ASRA practice advisory on local anesthetic systemic toxicity. Reg Anesth pain Med 2010;35(2):152–61.

41. Loftus RW, Koff MD, Birnbach DJ. The dynamics and implications of bacterial transmission events arising from the anesthesia work area. Anesth Analg 2015; 120(4):853–60.

42. Birnbach DJ, Rosen LF, Fitzpatrick M, et al. The use of a novel technology to study dynamics of pathogen transmission in the operating room. Anesth Analg 2015;120(4):844–7.

43. Birnbach DJ, Rosen LF, Fitzpatrick M, et al. A new approach to pathogen containment in the operating room: sheathing the laryngoscope after intubation. Anesth Analg 2015;121(5):1209–14.

44. Munoz-Price LS, Bowdle A, Johnston BL, et al. Infection prevention in the operating room anesthesia work area. Infect Control Hosp Epidemiol 2018;11:1–17.
45. Sobhy S, Zamora J, Dharmarajah K, et al. Anaesthesia-related maternal mortality in low-income and middle-income countries: a systematic review and meta-analysis. Lancet Glob Health 2016;4(5):e320–7.
46. Mhyre JM, Tsen LC, Einav S, et al. Cardiac arrest during hospitalization for delivery in the United States, 1998-2011. Anesthesiology 2014;120(4):810–8.
47. GBD 2015 Maternal Mortality Collaborators. Global, regional, and national levels of maternal mortality, 1990-2015: a systematic analysis for the Global Burden of Disease Study 2015. Lancet 2016;388(10053):1775–812.
48. Abir G, Mhyre J. Maternal mortality and the role of the obstetric anesthesiologist. Best Pract Res Clin Anaesthesiol 2017;31(1):91–105.
49. D'Angelo R, Smiley RM, Riley ET, et al. Serious complications related to obstetric anesthesia: the serious complication repository project of the Society for Obstetric Anesthesia and Perinatology. Anesthesiology 2014;120(6):1505–12.
50. Mhyre JM, Bateman BT. Stemming the tide of obstetric morbidity: an opportunity for the anesthesiologist to embrace the role of peridelivery physician. Anesthesiology 2015;123(5):986–9.
51. Bateman BT, Tsen LC. Anesthesiologist as epidemiologist: insights from registry studies of obstetric anesthesia-related complications. Anesthesiology 2014; 120(6):1311–2.
52. Mc QE, Leffert LR, Bateman BT. The role of the anesthesiologist in preventing severe maternal morbidity and mortality. Clin Obstet Gynecol 2018;61(2):372–86.
53. Reason J. Human error: models and management. BMJ 2000;320(7237):768–70.

Emerging Clinical Trends

Office Patient Safety

Roxane Gardner, MD, MSHPEd, DSc[a,b,c,d,*]

KEYWORDS

- Patient safety • Ambulatory care • Human factors • Diagnostic errors
- Safety culture • Disclosure and apology • Checklists • Simulation and drills

KEY POINTS

- Patient safety is the prevention of harm to patients and is indistinguishable from the delivery of quality care.
- Collaboration with human factors professionals engenders comprehensive analysis of impediments to safety and realistic, systematic solutions for clinical practice to ensure patient safety and quality of care.
- Diagnostic-related errors in the process of care are more problematic in outpatient settings, and a variety of factors contribute to their occurrence.
- Multiple strategies are needed to prevent or trap errors from harming patients in office practice, including a culture of patient safety, leadership whereby patient safety is a top priority, and instituting systems and mechanisms to ensure safety in office practice.
- Partnering with patients and including them in making office practice safer is essential for success.

INTRODUCTION

Safe office practice is a top priority for the American College of Obstetrics and Gynecology (ACOG). Douglas Kirkpatrick, in his inaugural speech as president of ACOG in 2008, announced that his first and foremost focus would be on patient safety.[1] He urged all members to use best practices for improving patient safety in office practice. Patient safety is the prevention of harm to patients, indistinguishable from the delivery of quality care.[2] Safety is the first domain of quality, thus inseparable.[3] The focus on safe patient care in the health professions came sharply into view with the Institute of Medicine's (IOM) landmark publication in 2001, "Crossing the Quality

[a] Obstetrics, Gynecology and Reproductive Biology, Harvard Medical School, Center for Medical Simulation, Boston, MA, USA; [b] Department of Obstetrics and Gynecology, Brigham and Women's Hospital, Center for Medical Simulation, Boston, MA, USA; [c] Division of Adolescent Gynecology, Boston Children's Hospital, 300 Longwood Avenue, 5th Floor, Boston, MA 02115, USA; [d] Center for Medical Simulation, Boston, MA, USA
* Division of Adolescent Gynecology, Boston Children's Hospital, 300 Longwood Avenue, 5th Floor, Boston, MA 02115.
E-mail address: rgardner1@bwh.harvard.edu

Chasm: A New Health System for the 21st Century."[3] The IOM articulated the need for a comprehensive transformation of the current health care delivery system in the United States with 6 domains of quality (**Table 1**).

ACOG acknowledged the importance of patient safety in the hospital setting and later broadened their advocacy for patient safety in ambulatory care and outpatient surgery settings.[4] This article explores factors that contribute to errors and patient harm in office practice, discusses key ways in which errors in the outpatient setting compare with those occurring in the inpatient setting, and describes strategies for supporting and improving patient safety in office practice. Patient safety in outpatient surgery settings are addressed separately in Mark S. DeFrancesco's article, "Patient Safety in Outpatient Procedures," in this issue.

HUMAN FACTORS AND CLINICAL PRACTICE

Human factors are "the study of the interrelationships between humans, the tools they use and the environments in which they live and work."[5] Human factors engineering encompasses the notion of human fallibility, the study of why errors happen, and how to obviate or prevent their occurrence. This involves examination of those elements that affect individuals, people, and their performance, including individual characteristics and environmental, organizational, and job-related circumstances; and thereafter designing systems that are resilient to unanticipated events.[6] Some common human factors categories include mental workload/cognition, perception, physical environment, physical demands, device/product design, process design, and teamwork. Veltman[7] highlighted some vexing issues and demands in clinical care that undermine safety and lower the risk for errors that cause patients harm (**Table 2**).

Application of human factors methodology to better understand safety problems in clinical care and design meaningful solutions to improve the delivery of health care has become increasingly more common.[8] The science of human factors will not provide instant solutions for improving health care.[9] However, collaboration with human factors professionals can render more comprehensive analysis of impediments to safety and engender realistic and systematic solutions for clinical practice-related issues to ensure patient safety and quality of care.

Table 1 Six domains of health care quality	
Safe	Avoiding harm to patients from care that is intended to help them
Effective	Providing services based on scientific knowledge to all who could benefit and refraining from providing services to those not likely to benefit (avoiding underuse and misuse, respectively)
Patient-centered	Providing care that is respectful and responsive to individual patient preferences, needs, and values, and ensuring that patient values guide all clinical decisions
Timely	Reducing waits and sometimes harmful delays for both those who receive and those who give care
Efficient	Avoiding waste, including waste of equipment, supplies, ideas, and energy
Equitable	Providing care that does not vary in quality because of personal characteristics such as gender, geographic location, and socioeconomic status

From Institute of Medicine (IOM). Crossing the quality chasm: a new health system for the 21st Century. Washington, DC: National Academy Press; 2001; with permission.

Table 2
Clinical care issues and demands that undermine safety

Issues and Demands	Example
Regional variation in clinical practice	• Deficient or inadequate guidelines, policies, or procedures • Lack of adherence to guidelines, policies, or procedures
Variation in clinical expertise	• Medical, surgical experience • Technical skills and abilities
Uncertainty	• Clinical presentation • Diagnosis • Decision making • Risk assessment • Management • Adherence to treatment • Response to treatment
Variation in resources	• Staff • Space • Equipment • Time
Presence demanded in more than one place at the same time	• Seeing patients in the office while managing an inpatient or postprocedure patient issue or a patient with a planned or unplanned emergency room visit
High clinical volume, largely normal patients	Busy office practice, mostly healthy patients and infrequently encountering high-acuity, complex patients
Growth in aging population with comorbidities	Older patient with high body mass index, hypertension, diabetes, and asthma who presents for vaginal bleeding
Off-site monitoring of high-risk clinical situations	Managing a busy office while directing care for a hospitalized or postprocedure patient
Frequent handoffs and inadequate sign-out	Multiple providers (physician assistant, nurse practitioner, clinician) managing patients of a primary provider who is away on vacation, conference, illness, or other personal matter
Protocols inadequate for referrals or consultations	Not knowing a patient missed or did not keep their specialty referral or consultation
Frequent interruptions and distractions	• Answering unexpected, urgent phone calls or questions from colleagues/staff, providers • Unexpected add-on urgent care or complex patient(s) to the day's schedule • Scheduled patient with acute issue
Critical decision making under stress	• Managing treatment/disposition of a complex patient during a busy, overbooked patient panel
Wishful thinking	• "Fallacy of the low-risk patient": continuing to perceive and manage a patient as low risk when their clinical circumstances now high risk
Fatigue, stress	• Being on-call and busy the night before • Family issue, such as managing a sick child or parent • Financial pressures • Personal illness or injury

(continued on next page)

Table 2 (continued)	
Issues and Demands	**Example**
Hierarchical systems	Organizing or ranking office staff and roles in a top-to-bottom structure, usually physicians being at the top
Poor teamwork and communication	• Lack of cooperation or coordination between staff and providers • Provider not listening to patient or staff about an issue • Staff or provider not speaking up about their concern(s)
Yielding to patient pressures	Patient requests for unnecessary medications or procedures
Overconfidence (hubris)	Presumption, arrogance in believing one is right in their determination or management plan and not entertaining alternative options

Data from Veltman LL. Getting to Havarti: moving toward patient safety in obstetrics. Obstet Gynecol 2007;110(5):1146–50.

SOURCES OF ERROR IN CLINICAL PRACTICE

Ambulatory care-related errors and adverse events differ from those related to hospital-based care. Analysis of malpractice claims data sheds light on such differences. In a retrospective analysis of malpractice claims paid on behalf of physicians between 2005 through 2009, originating in inpatient and outpatient settings 47.6% were for inpatient events and 43.1% were for events in the outpatient setting, and 9.4% involved events in both settings.[10] The number of claims significantly decreased from 2005 to 2009 for all 3 settings. However, the trend was greatest for the inpatient-setting events. The inpatient events were more commonly classified as related to surgery (34.1%), diagnosis (21.1%), and treatment (20.3%). By comparison, those events in outpatient settings were classified as related to diagnosis (45.9%), treatment (29.5%), and surgery (14.4%). Diagnostic-related errors in the process of care are more problematic in outpatient settings, and a variety of factors contribute to their occurrence. The Controlled Risk Insurance Company/Risk Management Foundation (CRICO/RMF) of the Harvard Medical Institutions regularly reviews malpractice data of the Harvard-affiliated hospitals. Using these data, LaValley[11] identified troublesome contributing factors for diagnostic errors in ambulatory care that included poor clinical judgment, poor clinical systems, inadequate communication between providers and between providers and patients, and inadequate documentation.[11] Clinical judgment comprises decision making and actions such as selection and management of treatment, patient assessment and history taking, physical evaluation of symptoms, and patient monitoring. Analysis of diagnostic errors in a large dataset of office-based malpractice claims identified similar findings, noting that 59% of such cases contained 3 or more contributing factors while few cases had only one.[12] CRICO/RMF analyzed comparative data for gynecologic malpractice claims from more than 20 states between 2004 and 2008[13] and found that of 472 cases, 241 were inpatients and 197 were outpatients while 34 were unclear as to location. Of the 197 outpatient cases, 88 (45%) were office-based and 81 (41%) were based in ambulatory surgery settings. Most office-based claims involved diagnostic errors (69%) and the rest involved medical treatment (15%), obstetric care (3%), communication (2%), medication (2%), and surgical treatment (2%). Issues among diagnostic errors included ordering of diagnostic or laboratory tests (52%), conducting a history or physical examination or evaluating symptoms (41%), and interpretation of tests (**Table 3**).

Final diagnosis for most of these diagnostic error-related claims involved cancer (48/61), primarily of the breast (n = 19), cervix (n = 11), uterus (n = 9), and ovary (n = 4). Only 4 of 61 cases involved a final diagnosis related to complications of pregnancy: ectopic (n = 3) and missed abortion (n = 1).[13] Using data from 3 studies of clinic-based primary care adults, the rate of diagnostic errors was 5.08%. Nationally this would affect 12 million patients annually.[14] Difficult to measure accurately, this rate is likely an underestimate. About half of these diagnostic errors could result in severe harm to patients.[15] Diagnostic errors in office practice constitute a serious matter involving multiple factors. No single strategy will obviate their occurrence.

STRATEGIES TO SUPPORT AND IMPROVE PATIENT SAFETY IN OFFICE PRACTICE

Multiple strategies are needed to prevent errors or mitigate harm in ambulatory settings. They include cultivating a culture of patient safety, providing consistent leadership, making patient safety a top priority, having a strong commitment to improve quality of care; and instituting systems and mechanisms to ensure safety in office practice.

Culture of Safety

The IOM defines safety culture as "an integrated pattern of individual and organizational behavior, based upon shared beliefs and values that continuously seeks to minimize patient harm that may result from the process of care delivery".[2] Cultivating a culture of safety in the office, regardless of specialty, is a key strategy for preventing or mitigating errors. The IOM believes that all health care settings should have comprehensive patient safety programs situated within a culture of safety.[2] One of the first steps toward creating a culture of safety is to acknowledge human fallibility. All members of the organization need to understand that humans are prone to error. Anyone working in bad systems can make errors. A safety culture environment is one in which members are accountable, respectful, and trustful toward each other; one in which errors or near misses can be reported free of shame and blame in an atmosphere of nonnegotiable mutual respect; and one in which all staff know clearly the

Table 3	
Risk-management issues identified in the diagnostic process of care	
Risk-Management Issues	**No. of Cases (%)**
History/physical and evaluation of symptoms	25 (41)
Order of diagnostic/lab tests	31 (52)
Performance of tests	1 (2)
Interpretation of tests	25 (41)
Receipt/transmittal of test results	10 (16)
Physician follow-up with patient	16 (26)
Referral management	9 (15)
Patient compliance with follow-up plan	9 (15)
Total	*61 (100)*

Data from Comparative benchmarking system. Cambridge (MA): CRICO/Risk Management Foundation of the Harvard Medical Institutions; 2010.

difference between acceptable and unacceptable behaviors. Errors and adverse events should be seen as opportunities to improve systems, not simply to punish a perpetrator. Dissecting what went wrong increases one's understanding of what measures can be created to prevent their occurrence. Conversely understanding "what went right" and creating systems that help "things go right" easily and consistently is equally important.[16]

A culture of safety cannot be mandated, it must be nurtured.[17] Desired behaviors must be nourished, encouraged, and proved successful to allow the culture to foster consistently safe, reliable care. The Institute for Healthcare Improvement supports assessment of the current culture as a fundamental first step toward improving ambulatory safety.[18] There are validated tools designed to query how staff perceive their environment and what needs improvement. The Agency for Healthcare Research and Quality (AHRQ) developed a patient safety culture instrument for use in office practice, the "Medical Office Survey on Patient Safety Culture."[19] The AHRQ advocates use of this survey for those offices having at least 3 clinicians who provide health care and prescribe medications. Smaller-sized office practices are encouraged to use the survey to promote conversations to improve patient safety. Assessing the status of safety can determine potential organizational, systemic, or individual issues for improvement. For practices with multiple sites, surveying each individually can provide comparisons and identify best practices for dissemination. Periodically readministering the survey is useful for evaluating the results of interventions over time.

Leadership

Quality and safety begins at the top, and this applies to managers, supervisors, or directors at every level of the organization. Leaders set the tone for organizational culture and acceptable behaviors in the office.[20] If the leader values patient safety as a primary concern and actively supports and promotes safety in the workplace, staff behavior will generally follow suit. Conversely, intimidating and disruptive behavior undermines a culture of safety, is unprofessional, and should not be tolerated regardless of who manifests such.[21] Disruptive behavior creates distress and lowers morale, whether the behavior is overt or passive-aggressive. Disruptive behavior is often shown by professionals in positions of power. It behooves all physicians, whether or not explicitly designated as leaders, to take personal responsibility for professionalism and be mindful of comments, gestures, or actions that may be construed as offensive to patients, staff, or colleagues.

Leadership in office safety includes establishing a system for reporting adverse events and near misses, including disruptive behaviors. Reporting systems should be confidential and staff should be confident that reporting and action(s) taken will engender meaningful change.[22,23] Systematic analysis of the reports by designated office staff to discern root causes and factors contributing to such events informs changes for safer care. A key to success in conducting such reviews is maintaining an open mind, avoiding a rush to judgment and assignment of blame. A successful reporting system includes feedback to staff. Feedback is essential to reinforce staff members' critical role at the front lines in detecting threats to safe patient care, ensuring their reporting translates into patient safety improvements. Leadership should explicitly identify who is responsible for programmatic changes and track such improvements. The sum total of this activity fosters a learning environment.[23]

In the event of error or adverse event, leaders should disclose to the patient, and their family as indicated, what happened. Ideally this is best when the facts are gathered and the situation investigated.[24,25] The more serious the event, the sooner disclosure should occur. Patients expect and want to know in a timely fashion what happened when things go wrong. They want acknowledgment of responsibility, empathy for what they have experienced, and an understanding of what will be done to prevent recurrence. Leadership needs to assist their staff, and colleagues involved or affected by the error may need support in managing the traumatic aftermath of emotions or physical deficits they may incur.[23,24] See Jonathan L. Gleason and colleagues' article, "Transparency and Disclosure," in this issue for a more detailed discussion.

Circumventing Diagnostic Errors in Office Practice

Diagnostic errors are problematic in ambulatory care. **Table 3** highlights a variety of issues arising in the process of care. Breakdowns and missteps commonly occur in the process of ordering, interpreting, and communicating test results, which facilitates missed or delayed diagnoses. Cognitive errors in clinical decision making and diagnosis are challenging to address and resolve.[26–29] Croskerry detailed more than 30 cognitive errors in diagnosis, including those associated with biases, failures in perception, and failures in heuristics.[29] Some of these are featured in **Table 4**.

Croskerry proposed a variety of strategies to overcome several of these biases, including developing insight/awareness, deliberately considering alternatives, metacognition or deliberately stepping back to reflect on the thinking process, decreasing

Table 4
Cognitive errors in diagnosis

Cognitive Error	Explanation
Availability bias	Tendency to assume, when judging possibilities or predicting outcomes, that the first possibility is selected as the most likely possibility: functioning as a cognitive "shortcut" in the setting of a complex situation
Confirmation bias	Tendency to focus on evidence that supports a working hypothesis without looking for further information that may refute the original hypothesis
Diagnosis momentum	Once a diagnosis is assigned, it is no longer a possibility but definite and all other possibilities are excluded
Framing effect	Being strongly influenced by how a problem is framed by patients, other providers, or staff
Fundamental attribution error	Tendency to be judgmental and blame patients for their problem
Order effects	Tendency to remember the beginning or end of information, but not all the information required during information transfer
Overconfidence bias	Tendency to think we know more than we do
Oversimplification of causality	Application of past events leads to underestimation of future consequences
Premature closure	
Thinking in causal series	Tendency for individuals within complex systems to think in linear sequences to form an immediate action without being aware of the "side effects" of that action to the system as a whole

Modified from Croskerry P. The importance of cognitive errors in diagnosis and strategies to minimize them. Acad Med 2003;78(8):775–80; with permission.

the reliance on memory, simulation (as in mental rehearsals or "cognitive walkthrough" for considering consequences of biases), cognitive forcing strategies (which help avoid specific predictable biases, making the task easier), minimizing time pressure, and feedback (rapid and reliable).

A systematic review of interventions aimed at reducing the likelihood of cognitive errors found a wide range of approaches, a few of which were tested and proven to work in actual clinical practice.[28] Interventions were organized into 3 general categories:

1. Increasing knowledge
2. Improving clinical reasoning
3. Getting help from colleagues, consultants, or tools

Disease-specific training seemed to be the intervention best supported for increasing knowledge. However, the use of simulation for teaching clinicians about diagnostic errors and practicing ways to prevent them seemed promising. Feedback was also deemed important for reducing overconfidence, helping clinicians appreciate the possibility of their errors and trying to avoid them. Reflective practice and active metacognitive review offered the greatest potential to improve clinical reasoning by minimizing premature closure, framing bias and context-based errors. Decision-support tools are practical and can be implemented system wide. These tools must be functional, efficient, and readily accessible, and clinicians must be willing to use them. Meanwhile, obtaining help via consultations and second opinions brings new perspectives by. The investigators supported more rigorous evaluation of interventions aimed at preventing cognitive errors and advocated for more research in this area.

Office-based systems for managing test results, consults/referrals, and patient transfers/transmission of information and follow-up between providers and patient-provider should be consistent, efficient, timely, and effective. Such systems may be electronic, paper-based log books, or spreadsheets. However, adoption of electronic health record (EHR) technology has grown significantly since passage of the American Recovery and Reinvestment Act of 2009, providing incentives to promote meaningful use.[30] EHRs currently available typically integrate result management tools or tracking systems to aid clinicians in follow-up of critical tests or referrals. Further improvement is needed to promote interoperability between different EHR systems. Whether tracking or management systems are paper-based or computer-based, it is essential to maintain vigilance for missing or incomplete information. ACOG provides additional guidance and resources for developing tracking and reminder systems.[31]

EHRs are helpful mechanisms for decreasing reliance on memory. In addition, standardization of clinical management or procedures,[32] coupled with the use of checklists or cognitive aids, are exceptionally helpful.[33] These tools are ideal for promoting standardized processes and confirming that the team performs all the proper steps.

Team-based approaches to minimizing cognitive errors in the office include implementing staff huddles or briefings. Ideally these take place at the beginning of the day or before each office session, and provide opportunities to facilitate explicit communication and a shared mental model about patient appointments and patient flow. Explicit sharing of information allows staff to better anticipate the needs of patients and their providers, be prepared for clinical issues that may arise during the day, and stay vigilant as the day evolves.[34–36] Tracking lessons learned from these daily huddles can be reviewed at weekly or monthly staff meetings and further support organizational learning and safety culture.

Medication Errors

Medication-related errors in office gynecology that harm patients occur less frequently than diagnostic errors. Adverse drug events and medication safety are among the most studied topics in safety-related outpatient research.[37] EHRs are exceptionally helpful for ensuring that the correct medications and dosages are ordered for the appropriate patients; and relayed directly to the pharmacy free of transcription errors.[38,39] The ACOG supports broad-based strategies for improving medication safety, including the use of health information technology, computerized order entry by physicians, and electronic prescribing.[40] ACOG also strongly advocates for patient involvement, including patient education and shared decision making to improve adherence to treatment regimens, outcomes, and patient satisfaction, and understanding of proper usage. Especially when electronic systems are not available, strategies to improve medication safety include accurate documentation, medication reconciliation, legible writing, using zeros and decimal points appropriately, avoiding nonstandardized abbreviations, minimizing reliance on verbal orders, and ensuring patient involvement.

Partnering with Patients

Providing care that is respectful and responsive to individual patient preferences, needs, and values, and ensuring that patient values guide all clinical decisions, is the third domain of quality.[3] This is the cornerstone of patient-centered care as defined by the IOM.[3] Patients are central and fundamental to the provision of health care services. Patient-centered care involves respect for patients' values, preferences, and expressed needs; coordinated and seamless integration of care; providing accurate and complete information in understandable language and terminology; attention to the impact of physical ailments and provision of comfort; provision of emotional support; and involvement of family and friends as per patient preferences. The ACOG promotes actively involving patients in planning and delivering health care services as a means of improving safety and quality of care.[41] Increasing patient engagement helps to reduce the risk of adverse events and improve patient outcomes, satisfaction, and adherence to treatment. A scoping review of patient-centered care found that achieving effective communication, partnership, and health promotion are critical to improving outcomes.[42] Creating an atmosphere that fosters patient engagement and mindfulness of health literacy, and that facilitates patients speaking about their concerns and misunderstandings, will contribute greatly toward improving the patient experience in office practice and mitigation of errors[43] (see Stephanie K. Sargent and Richard Waldman's article, "The Patient Experience and Safety," in this issue).

Simulation/Office Drills

Simulations or office drills provide unique opportunities for staff to practice managing infrequent, high-acuity events and better prepare them for the real situation. Simulations can be conducted in several ways, including table-top walk-throughs, role-playing, or using mannequins. High-fidelity mannequins, full-body human patient simulators, can also be used but may not be practical or affordable in smaller office settings or remote locations. Regardless of the technology selected for the drill, it is crucial to set aside time to debrief with the team and discuss what went well and what could be done to respond better in the next drill or real situation. Topics to consider for office drills are listed in **Box 1**.

Emergencies happen at unexpected times and locations, so it is critical to be prepared. Clinicians and office staff should think about how they would respond. Consider designating emergency response roles for certain individuals. Everyone

---

Box 1
Suggestions for office drills

- Vasovagal episode
- Precipitous vaginal delivery
- Reaction to local anesthetic
- Cardiorespiratory arrest
- Unexpected hemorrhage during procedure
  - Vulvar
  - Vaginal
  - Cervical
  - Uterine
  - Limb (implant-related)
- Excessive sedation
- Opioid overdose
- Allergic reaction/anaphylaxis
- Patient or staff injury
  - Fall
  - Laceration
  - Contamination
- Upset patient or family member
- Fire
- Power failure
- Chemical spill
- Active shooter

---

should be familiar with key life-saving equipment, such as the automated external defibrillator, fire alarm locations, or hotline if one exists. The ACOG strongly supports simulations and drills for both inpatient and outpatient settings.[44–46]

SUMMARY

Patient safety in the ambulatory setting is integral to providing high-quality patient care. Patient safety does not just happen: it requires leadership, time, thoughtful attention, and deliberate practice. A culture of patient safety nourished by strong, consistent leadership facilitates discussion and learning from what went wrong and what went well, and constantly strives to improve processes and procedures benefiting patients and staff. Professional societies support efforts to establish and maintain patient safety in office practice, providing practical tools to facilitate patient safety in all aspects of office-based care. Some of these tools and techniques have been reviewed in this article and, it is hoped, will stimulate curiosity and further exploration about what else may bolster safety in the office setting. Patient safety is a journey and a priority for all clinicians. We must all strive for excellence in the provision of safe patient care in our everyday office and hospital activities. Our patients and our colleagues deserve no less.

REFERENCES

1. New president to focus on patient safety. ACOG Today 2008;52(6). 1 & 14. Available at: https://www.acog.org/-/media/ACOG-Today/acogToday0708.pdf?dmc=1&ts=20180925T2040447417. Accessed September 25, 2018.

2. Erickson SM, Wolcott J, Corrigan JM, et al, editors. Patient safety: achieving a new standard for care. Washington, DC: National Academies Press; 2004.

3. Briere R. Crossing the quality chasm: a new health system for the 21st century. National Academies Press; 2001. Washington, DC.

4. Purdon TF. Caring. Obstet Gynecol 2001;98(4):545–9.

5. Weinger MB, Pantiskas C, Wiklund M, et al. Incorporating human factors in the design of medical devices. JAMA 1998;280(17):1484.

6. Russ AL, Fairbanks RJ, Karsh BT, et al. The science of human factors: separating fact from fiction. BMJ Qual Saf 2013;22(10):802–8.

7. Veltman L. Getting to Havarti. Obstet Gynecol 2007;110(5):1146–50.

8. Carayon P, Xie A, Kianfar S. Human factors and ergonomics as a patient safety practice. BMJ Qual Saf 2014;23:196–205.

9. Shouhed D, Gerwertz B, Wiegmann D, et al. Integrating human factors research and surgery. Arch Surg 2012;147(12):1141–6.

10. Bishop TJ, Ryan AM, Casalino LP. Paid malpractice claims for adverse events in inpatient and outpatient settings. JAMA 2011;305(23):2427–31.

11. LaValley D. Office-based malpractice cases 1997-2006. Forum 2007;25(2):1–2.

12. Gandhi TK, Kachalia A, Thomas EJ, et al. Missed and delayed diagnoses in the ambulatory setting: a study of closed malpractice claims. Ann Intern Med 2006; 145:488–96.

13. CRICO Strategies. Comparative benchmarking system [database]. Cambridge (MA): CRICO/Risk Management Foundation of the Harvard Medical Institutions; 2010.

14. Singh H, Meyer AND, Thomas EJ. The frequency of diagnostic errors in outpatient care: estimations from three large observational studies involving US adult populations. BMJ Qual Saf 2014;23:727–31.

15. Singh H, Giardina TD, Meyer AN, et al. Types and origins of diagnostic errors in primary care settings. JAMA Intern Med 2013;173(6):418–25.

16. Hollnagel E, Wears RL, Braithwaite J. From Safety-I to Safety-II: a white paper. Odense, Gainesville, Sydney: The resilient health care net: University of Southern Denmark, University of Florida, Macquarie University; 2015.

17. Carroll JS, Quijada MA. Redirecting traditional professional values to support safety: changing organisational culture in health care. BMJ Qual Saf 2004; 13(suppl 2):ii16–21.

18. Gandhi T. 3 tips for getting started on ambulatory safety. Improvement blog. Boston (MA): Institute for Healthcare Improvement; 2018. Available at: http://www.ihi.org/communities/blogs/3-tips-for-getting-started-on-ambulatory-safety. Accessed September 22, 2018.

19. Agency for Healthcare Research and Quality. US Department of Health and Human Services. Surveys on patient safety culture. Available at: https://www.ahrq.gov/sops/index.html. Accessed September 13, 2018.

20. Gluck P. Physician leadership: essential in creating a culture of safety. Clin Obstet Gynecol 2010;53(3):473–81.

21. Committee on Patient Safety and Quality Improvement. Committee Opinion No. 683: behavior that undermines a culture of safety. Obstet Gynecol 2017;129: e1–4.

22. Gandhi TK, Graydon-Baker E, Huber CN, et al. Closing the loop: follow-up and feedback in a patient safety program. Jt Comm J Qual Patient Saf 2005;31(11): 614–21.

23. Ginsburg LR, Chuang YT, Berta WB, et al. The relationship between organizational leadership for safety and learning from patient safety events. Health Serv Res 2010;45(3):607–32.

24. Wu AW. Medical error: the second victim: the doctor who makes the mistake needs help too. Br Med J 2000;320(7237):726.

25. Burlison JD, Scott SD, Browne EK, et al. The second victim experience and support tool: validation of an organizational resource for assessing second victim effects and the quality of support resources. J Patient Saf 2017;13(2):93–102.

26. Graber M, Gordon R, Franklin N. Reducing diagnostic errors in medicine: what's the goal? Acad Med 2002;77:981–92.

27. Elstein AS, Schwarz A. Clinical problem solving and diagnostic decision making: selective review of the cognitive literature. BMJ 2002;324:729–32.

28. Graber ML, Kissam S, Payne VL, et al. Cognitive interventions to reduce diagnostic error: a narrative review. BMJ Qual Saf 2012;21(7):535–57.

29. Crosberry P. The importance of cognitive errors in diagnosis and strategies to minimize them. Acad Med 2003;78:775–80.

30. Eisenberg M, Hom J, Sharp C. The electronic health record as a healthcare management strategy and implications for obstetrics and gynecologic practice. Curr Opin Obstet Gynecol 2013;25(6):476–81.

31. Committee on Patient Safety and Quality Improvement, American College of Obstetricians and Gynecologists. Committee Opinion No. 546: tracking and reminder systems. Obstet Gynecol 2012;120:1535–7.

32. Committee on Patient Safety and Quality Improvement. Committee Opinion No. 629: clinical guidelines and standardization of practice to improve outcomes. Obstet Gynecol 2015;125:1027–9.

33. American College of Obstetricians and Gynecologists' Committee on Patient Safety and Quality Improvement. Committee Opinion No. 680: the use and development of checklists in obstetrics and gynecology. Obstet Gynecol 2016;128:e237–40.

34. Houck S. What works: effective tools and case studies to improve clinical office practice. Boulder (CO): Health Press Publishing; 2004.

35. Stewart EE, Johnson BC. Huddles: improve office efficiency in mere minutes daily gatherings of your care team can help you meet daily challenges. Fam Pract Manag 2007;14(6):27–9.

36. Institute for Healthcare Improvement. Balance supply and demand on a daily, weekly, and long-term basis: use regular huddles and staff meetings to plan production and to optimize team communication. Available at: http://www.ihi.org/resources/Pages/Changes/UseRegularHuddlesandStaffMeetingstoPlanProductionandtoOptimizeTeamCommunication.aspx. Accessed October 2, 2018.

37. Gandhi TK, Weingart SN, Borus J, et al. Adverse drug events in ambulatory care. N Engl J Med 2003;348(16):1556–64.

38. American Academy of Pediatrics Council on Clinical Information Technology, Gerstle RS. Electronic prescribing systems in pediatrics: the rationale and functionality requirements. Pediatrics 2007;119(6):1229–31.

39. Centers for Medicare and Medicaid Services. Electronic Prescribing (eRx) Incentive Program. Available at: https://www.cms.gov/ERXIncentive/. Accessed October 2, 2018.

40. Committee on Patient Safety and Quality Improvement. Committee opinion no. 531: improving medication safety. Obstet Gynecol 2012;120:406–10.

41. American College of Obstetricians and Gynecologists Committee on Patient Safety and Quality Improvement. ACOG Committee Opinion No. 490: partnering with patients to improve safety. Obstet Gynecol 2011;117:1247–9.

42. Constand MK, MacDermid JC, Dal Bello-Haas V, et al. Scoping review of patient-centered care approaches in healthcare. BMC Health Serv Res 2014;14:271.

43. Fisher KA, Smith KM, Gallagher TH, et al. We want to know: patient comfort speaking up about breakdowns in care and patient experience. BMJ Qual Saf 2018. https://doi.org/10.1136/bmjqs-2018-008159.

44. American College of Obstetricians and Gynecologists, Women's Health Care Physicians; [Committee on Patient Safety and Quality Improvement]. Quality and safety in women's health care. 2nd edition. Washington, DC: American College of Obstetricians and Gynecologists; 2010.

45. Erickson TB, Kirkpatrick DH, DeFrancesco MS, et al. Executive summary of the American College of Obstetricians and Gynecologists Presidential Task Force on Patient Safety in the Office Setting: reinvigorating safety in office-based gynecologic surgery. Obstet Gynecol 2010;115:147–51.

46. American College of Obstetricians and Gynecologists Committee on Patient Safety and Quality Improvement. Preparing for clinical emergencies in obstetrics and gynecology. Committee Opinion No. 590. Obstet Gynecol 2014;123:722–5.

Applying Patient Safety to Reduce Maternal Mortality

Caitlin Baptiste, MD[a],*, Mary E. D'Alton, MD[b]

KEYWORDS

- Patient safety tools • Bundles • Early warning systems
- Maternal morbidity and mortality • Racial disparities

KEY POINTS

- Maternal early warning systems provide an opportunity for early intervention to prevent maternal morbidity and mortality.
- Patient care bundles help implement evidence-based practices into routine care.
- Standardizing care decreases patient care variation and improves patient safety.
- Monitoring outcomes through root cause analysis is imperative to improving outcomes.

INTRODUCTION

The maternal mortality rate in the Unites States has not decreased in more than 2 decades and now may be increasing.[1,2] The Unites States is an outlier among other developed countries regarding the rate of maternal mortality. The Centers for Disease Control and Prevention (CDC) published the Report from Nine Maternal Mortality Review Committees and found that nearly 50% of all pregnancy-related deaths were caused by hemorrhage, cardiovascular and coronary conditions, cardiomyopathies, and infection, and that more than 60% of these pregnancy-related deaths are preventable.[3] The numbers are a major concern but also provide opportunity for action and improvement. This article explores the patient safety tools that have been developed to reduce maternal morbidity and mortality.

EARLY WARNING ALERT SYSTEMS AND TRIGGERS

Knowing that most maternal morbidity and mortality is preventable, many local, state, and national projects have investigated when and how to reduce the number of women from dying from childbirth.[2–5] Reviews of maternal mortality cases showing

Disclosure Statement: None.
[a] Maternal Fetal Medicine, Department of Obstetrics and Gynecology, Columbia University Irving Medical Center, 622 West 168th Street, PH 16-28, New York, NY 10032, USA;
[b] Department of Obstetrics and Gynecology, Columbia University Irving Medical Center, 622 West 168th Street, PH 16-66, New York, NY 10032, USA
* Corresponding author.
E-mail address: cb2670@cumc.columbia.edu

Obstet Gynecol Clin N Am 46 (2019) 353–365
https://doi.org/10.1016/j.ogc.2019.01.016
0889-8545/19/© 2019 Elsevier Inc. All rights reserved.

obgyn.theclinics.com

that women have abnormal vital signs before decompensating lead to the development of early warning systems. This critical window provides an opportunity for earlier intervention.[6]

Other specialties have implemented early warning systems; however, many of the existing alert systems are not applicable to obstetric patients.[7,8] For example, the systemic inflammatory response (SIRS) criteria and the modified early warning system (MEWS), used in general medicine patients to predict sepsis, were not applicable in obstetric patients with intrauterine infection. Sixty-three percent of women with chorioamnionitis met SIRS criteria; however, there was only a 0.9% positive predictive value for sepsis. Ten percent of women with chorioamnionitis had a positive MEWS score with only a 0.05% positive predictive value for sepsis.[9]

Subsequently, the Sequential Organ Failure Assessment (SOFA) score or the quick-SOFA (qSOFA) score was developed to identify patients at risk of dying from sepsis. The qSOFA score has 3 components that are readily identifiable at the bedside: respiratory rate (>22/min), altered mentation, and a systolic blood pressure less than 110 mm Hg. Patients with qSOFA scores of 2 or higher have a 3-fold to 14-fold increase in hospital mortality compared with those with score less than 2.[8] With normal physiologic changes, many healthy pregnant women have systolic blood pressure less than 110 mm Hg. This would give them at least 1 point on the qSOFA score, negating its validity.

Early warning systems made for general medical patients may falsely highlight normal physiologic changes in pregnancy, but also do not capture the fact that pregnant women die from causes that are different from causes in general medical patients. In the 2013 National Hospital Discharge Survey from the CDC, the top causes of death in hospitalized patients were respiratory failure, pneumonitis, and septicemia.[10] Obstetric patients die from hemorrhage, cardiopulmonary dysfunction, preeclampsia-hypertension, and sepsis.

Early warning systems unique to obstetric patients have been created due to the physiologic changes that occur in pregnancy and the relatively short list of conditions responsible for most maternal morbidity and mortality.

In 2007, the United Kingdom recommended adoption of the Modified Early Obstetric Warning System (MEOWS). In the MEOWS system, 2 moderately abnormal parameters (yellow alert) or 1 severely abnormal parameter (red alert) requires a provider to assess the patient and make a plan. The parameters used in the MEOW scoring system include vital signs, pain score, and neurologic response.[11] Studies have evaluated the validity of the MEOWS. The data demonstrate a sensitivity of 89% and a specificity of 79% for identifying morbidity from hemorrhage, hypertensive disease of pregnancy, and suspected infection.[11]

In 2010, the Joint Commission required birthing facilities to develop early warning signs indicating a change or deterioration in a patient's clinical status. Further evaluation by a provider would be required if positive.[5] The National Partnership for Maternal Safety, an effort composed of leaders from organizations across the spectrum of women's health care, including hospital organizations, various states, and regulatory bodies, met in 2012 to develop a structured approach for recognition of early warning signs and symptoms.[3] The National Partnership for Maternal Safety proposed a simplified early warning system, the Maternal Early Warning Criteria (MEWC). In the MEWC system, if the patient has any single, confirmed, abnormal parameter, a provider is asked to assess the patient at the bedside.[6] The American College of Obstetricians and Gynecologists (ACOG) District II's Safe Motherhood Initiative endorsed use of MEWC for all hospitals providing obstetric care in New York.

Despite widespread support of early warning criteria, data are lacking as to what degree of abnormality should trigger evaluation and intervention. The key aspects to any successful maternal early warning system include the following[12]:

1. Identifying patients at risk for critical illness and who benefit from timely intervention
2. Promptly reporting abnormal parameters
3. Bedside evaluation by a provider when abnormal parameters are reported
4. Minimizing false-positives to avoid alarm fatigue and desensitization

In 2016, Shields and colleagues[13] developed a 2-tiered Maternal Early Warning Trigger (MEWT) tool system. One single severe abnormal value or 2 nonsevere abnormal values were required to trigger a warning. The tool addressed the 4 most common areas of maternal morbidity, including sepsis, cardiopulmonary dysfunction, preeclampsia-hypertension, and hemorrhage. They piloted the tool in 6 of 29 hospitals within a large hospital system. There were more than 30,000 deliveries at the pilot sites and 140,000 deliveries at the nonpilot sites. Use of the MEWT tool resulted in significant reductions in severe maternal morbidity as defined by the CDC.

Table 1 compares the MEOWS, MEWT, and MEWC, the 3 early warning systems discussed previously. The MEOWS and the MEWT stratify parameters into 2 categories requiring a more comprehensive assessment before reporting abnormalities. At the authors' institution, the MEWC system is used to simplify the initial assessment in an attempt to capture all at-risk patients and intervene in a timely manner.

Despite their promise to identify patients at risk for decompensation, among the several proposed trigger systems, evidence is limited on which is superior, and alert fatigue among providers is a rising concern[14] (https://www.ecri.org). Although these scoring systems may accurately predict adverse outcomes or death in patients admitted to intensive care units, the overall impact on health outcomes and resource utilization remains unclear.[15] Optimizing alert system performance is imperative, as a warning system that leads to a large number of false-positives may actually worsen clinical care. False alarms quickly become a nuisance and providers become desensitized to their limited clinical value.

BUNDLES

The Institute for Healthcare Improvement defines a bundle as a small set of evidence-based practices, generally 3 to 5, that, when performed collectively and reliably, improve patient outcomes.[16] Funded in 2006, The California Maternal Quality Care Collaborative (CMQCC), an organization committed to ending preventable morbidity and mortality in maternity care, put forth patient safety bundles. With more than 200 participating hospitals in the CMQCC, the maternal mortality rate in California declined by 55% between 2006 and 2013 (See Cathie Markow and Elliott K. Main's article, "Creating change at scale: Quality Improvement Strategies used by the California Maternal Quality Care Collaborative," in this issue). The Alliance for Innovation on Maternal Health (AIM) is a national data-driven maternal safety and quality improvement initiative. Both AIM and the CMQCC have worked with ACOG's Council on Patient Safety in Women's Healthcare to disseminate patient safety bundles. There are currently established patient safety bundles focusing on obstetric hemorrhage, severe hypertension, and venous thromboembolism (https://safehealthcareforeverywoman);[3] however, there are many other aspects of obstetric care that lend themselves to bundled care.

Obstetric Hemorrhage

Obstetric hemorrhage is a leading cause of maternal death worldwide.[17] In 2012, Clark and Hankins[18] shared 10 clinical diamonds to prevent maternal death, 5 of which were

Table 1
Maternal early warning systems

	Modified Early Obstetric Warning System (MEOWS) Singh et al,[11] 2012. Trigger: One Red or 2 Yellow Values		Maternal Early Warning Criteria (MEWC) Mhyre et al,[6] 2014. Trigger: One, Confirmed Value		Maternal Early Warning Trigger (MEWT) Shields et al,[13] 2016. Trigger: One Severe or 2 Nonsevere Values, Sustained for >20 min	
	Red	Yellow			Severe	Nonsevere
Temperature (degrees celsius)	<35 or >38	35–36	Systolic BP, mm Hg	<90 or >160	Maternal heart rate >130 beats per min	Temperature >38 or <36 celsius
Systolic BP, mm Hg	<90 or >160	150–160 or 90–100	Diastolic BP, mm Hg	>100	Respiratory rate >30 breaths/min	BP >160/110 or <85/45 mm Hg
Diastolic BP, mm Hg	>100	90–100	Heart rate beats per min	<50 or >120	Mean arterial pressure <55 mm Hg	Heart rate >110 or <50 beats per min
Heart rate, beats per min	<40 or >120	100–120 or 40–50	Respiratory rate, breaths per min	<10 or >30	Oxygen saturation <90% or nurse concern	Respiratory rate >34 or <10 per minute
Respiratory rate, breaths per min	<10 or >30	21–30	Oxygen saturation on room air at sea level, %	<95		Oxygen saturation >93%
Oxygen saturation, %	<95	<95	Oliguria, mL/h for >2 h	<35		Fetal heart rate >160
Pain score	2 or 3		Maternal agitation, confusion or unresponsiveness	Present		Altered mental status
Neurologic response	Unresponsive, pain	Voice	Patient with preeclampsia reporting a nonremitting headache or shortness of breath	Present		Disproportionate pain

Three different obstetric early warning systems, each of which use varying signs and symptoms with various cutoff points to identify patients at risk.
Abbreviation: BP, blood pressure.
Data from Refs.[6,11,13]

related to hemorrhage.[18] Hemorrhage is not a diagnosis but a symptom of many different diagnoses with several different treatments. Regardless of the etiology, most maternal deaths due to hemorrhage are preventable.[19] The various errors include underestimating blood loss, inattention to signs of hemorrhage and hypovolemia, failure to act decisively, and failure to transfuse blood products in a timely manner. Basically there is often denial and delay.[3]

The Council on Patient Safety, ACOG, and AIM recommend that hospitals providing obstetric care have an established hemorrhage protocol, event checklist, and hemorrhage supply kit readily available.[3,20] The bundle is organized into 4 areas: *readiness, recognition and prevention, response and reporting,* and *systems learning.* Every unit must be *ready* with supplies, checklists, and instruction cards; access to medications; adequate providers; and the ability to use a massive transfusion protocol. Providers must *recognize* the risk for hemorrhage for each patient, quantify blood loss, and actively manage the third stage of labor. To *respond,* every obstetric unit must have escalating obstetric hemorrhage management plans and support systems in place for patients, families, and staff. And perhaps most importantly, a culture of *reporting and improvement* must be established. After every hemorrhage, a postevent debrief and multidisciplinary review will allow units to monitor outcomes and improve future care. (https:// safehealthcareforeverywoman.org/patient-safety-bundles/obstetric-hemorrhage/) is the obstetric hemorrhage bundle provided by the Council on Patient Safety.

Severe Hypertension in Pregnancy

Hypertensive disorders of pregnancy contribute greatly to maternal morbidity and mortality. Up to 60% of maternal deaths due to hypertension are potentially preventable.[3,19,21] Blood pressure control can prevent hemorrhagic stroke and cerebral infarction. Sequelae of hypertension occur for several reasons including inadequate treatment, failure to recognize HELLP (hemolysis, elevated liver enzymes, and low platelet count) syndrome, and failure to recognize and treat pulmonary edema.[22]

Electronic order sets and standardized algorithms have been developed for managing severe hypertension in pregnancy. ACOG District II's Safe Motherhood Initiative (**Fig. 1**) and the Council on Patient Safety have published checklists and bundles for the management of severe hypertension. Similar to hemorrhage, the bundle is categorized into 4 domains: *readiness, recognition and prevention, response and reporting,* and *systems learning.* The bundle recommends notification of a physician or primary provider if the systolic blood pressure is >160 mm Hg or diastolic blood pressure is >110 mm Hg for 2 measurements within 15 minutes. After the second elevated reading, treatment should be initiated as soon as possible within 30 to 60 minutes of confirmed severe hypertension.

Algorithms are available to help with the use of intravenous (IV) labetalol, IV hydralazine, and oral nifedipine[23] The ACOG Committee Opinion from 2017 highlights that the use of IV labetalol, IV hydralazine, or immediate-release oral nifedipine does not require cardiac monitoring or transfer of care to another unit. Personnel in all hospital settings, including antepartum, postpartum, and the emergency room, should be able to provide these initial medications.[23] In hospitals without immediate physician availability, nursing and advance practitioners should be comfortable using the protocols to administer first-line antihypertensive while awaiting the arrival of the physician.

Venous Thromboembolism Bundle

In a review of hospital-based maternal deaths, venous thromboembolism (VTE) was found to be the single cause of mortality most amenable to improvement by systemic changes in practice.[22] The World Health Organization found embolism to be responsible

EXAMPLE

Hypertensive Emergency Checklist

HYPERTENSIVE EMERGENCY:

- Two severe BP values (≥160/110) taken 15–60 min apart. Values do not need to be consecutive.
- May treat within 15 min if clinically indicated

☐ Call for Assistance

☐ Designate:
  ○ Team leader
  ○ Checklist reader/recorder
  ○ Primary RN

☐ Ensure side rails up

☐ Ensure medications appropriate given patient history

☐ Administer seizure prophylaxis (magnesium sulfate first line agent, unless contraindicated)

☐ Antihypertensive therapy within 1 hour for persistent severe range BP

☐ Place IV; Draw preeclampsia labs

☐ Antenatal corticosteroids (if <34 wk of gestation)

☐ Re-address VTE prophylaxis requirement

☐ Place indwelling urinary catheter

☐ Brain imaging if unremitting headache or neurological symptoms

☐ Debrief patient, family, and obstetric team

† "Active asthma" is defined as:
  Ⓐ symptoms at least once a wk, or
  Ⓑ use of an inhaler, corticosteroids for asthma during the pregnancy, or
  Ⓒ any history of intubation or hospitalization for asthma.

Magnesium Sulfate

Contraindications: Myasthenia gravis; avoid with pulmonary edema, use caution with renal failure

IV access:
☐ Load 4-6 grams 10% magnesium sulfate in 100 mL solution over 20 min
☐ Label magnesium sulfate; Connect to labeled infusion pump
☐ Magnesium sulfate maintenance 1-2 grams/hour

No IV access:
☐ 10 grams of 50% solution IM (5 g in each buttock)

Antihypertensive Medications

For SBP ≥160 or DBP ≥110
(See SMI algorithms for complete management when necessary to move to another agent after 2 doses.)

☐ **Labetalol** (initial dose: 20mg); Avoid parenteral labetalol with active asthma, heart disease, or congestive heart failure; use with caution with history of asthma

☐ **Hydralazine** (5–10mg IV* over 2 min); May increase risk of maternal hypotension

☐ **Oral Nifedipine** (10 mg capsules); Capsules should be administered orally, not punctured or otherwise administered sublingually

* *Maximum cumulative IV-administered doses should not exceed 220 mg labetalol or 25 mg hydralazine in 24 ho*

Note: *If first line agents unsuccessful, emergency consult with specialist (MFM, internal medicine, OB anesthesiology, critical care) is recommended*

Anticonvulsant Medications

For recurrent seizures or when magnesium sulfate contraindicated

☐ **Lorazepam (Ativan):** 2–4 mg IV x 1, may repeat once after 10–15 min
☐ **Diazepam (Valium):** 5–10 mg IV q 5–10 min to maximum dose 30 mg

Safe Motherhood Initiative

Revised January 2019

Fig. 1. ACOG District II's safe motherhood initiative severe hypertension checklist available online and via the safe motherhood initiative phone app. (*From* American College of Obstetricians and Gynecologists. Women's Health Care Physicians. District II: Severe Hypertension; with permission. Available at: https://www.acog.org/-/media/Districts/District-II/Public/SMI/v2/19sm01a170703HTEmrgncyCheck1.pdf?dmc=1&ts=20190212T1429306115.)

for 14.9% of maternal deaths in developed nations.[24] There are 2 populations at risk of developing VTE:

1. Women delivered by cesarean
2. Women with a history of significant risk factors for VTE during and after pregnancy

There are several different guidelines regarding thromboprophylaxis for women undergoing cesarean delivery. The Joint Commission recommends sequential compression devices for patients undergoing cesarean delivery and chemoprophylaxis with low-molecular-weight heparin (LMWH) for patients at high risk for VTE postpartum. With the increase in maternal medical comorbidities and rates of obesity, there is a compelling argument for routine VTE prophylaxis.

The ACOG does not recommend VTE prophylaxis for all women who undergo a cesarean delivery; only those with a high risk for VTE.[25] The Royal College of Obstetricians and Gynecologists (RCOG) recommends that all women who undergo cesarean deliveries should be considered for thromboprophylaxis with LMWH for 10 days after delivery, and for those with additional risk factors, the LMWH should be continued for 6 weeks postpartum. After considering recommendations from ACOG, RCOG, the American College of Chest Physicians, and the American Society of Regional Anesthesia and Pain Medicine, ACOG District II Safe Motherhood Initiative developed a VTE Bundle. This bundle recommends that all patients be assessed for VTE risk during their initial prenatal visit, during any antepartum hospitalization, during labor and delivery, and postpartum at discharge. Specifically for women who have undergone a cesarean delivery, prophylaxis is recommended in the hospital. They may either receive empiric pharmacologic prophylaxis in the absence of a contraindication or may receive prophylaxis based on risk factors.[26] **Table 2** compares the various recommendations regarding VTE prophylaxis after cesarean delivery.

Implementing and Individualizing Bundled Care

Despite best efforts, implementing the hemorrhage bundle is often difficult given the various etiologies of hemorrhage and its sometimes-rapid onset. Every bundle developed by the Council for Patient Safety is available for free download at safehealthcareforeverywoman.org, and ACOG District II and the Safe Motherhood Initiative have a phone app that is free and provides the bundles as well as other useful resources. The authors recommend the use of these resources. The goal of bundle implementation is not to memorize all possible contingencies but to use checklists and resources to standardize care.

Bundles provide a structured approach to commonly seen obstetric emergencies; however, there is room for individualization.[27] For example, methylergonovine maleate should be avoided in women with hypertension, as it may further increase blood pressure. Most clinicians know that prostaglandins such as carboprost should not be given to patients with asthma. There are several other classes of drugs that may also cause bronchospasm, such as the beta-blocker labetalol. For these medications, the benefits of treatment must be carefully weighed against potential risks in pregnant patients with asthma.[27] Although standardized care improves outcomes, the provider must individually assess each patient before using a treatment bundle. The clinician must consider potential medical problems, medication interactions, or allergies.

STANDARDIZATION OF PRACTICE

Improved standardization and communication through the use of protocols and checklists has been shown to reduce patient harm.[28] ACOG endorses the use of

Table 2 Differing recommendations for thromboprophylaxis after cesarean delivery			
	American College of Obstetricians and Gynecologists ACOG Practice Bulletin, July 2018	Royal College of Obstetricians and Gynecologists RCOG, April 2015	National Partnership for Maternal Safety/Safe Motherhood Initiative Anesthesia-Analgesia, October 2016
Pneumatic Compression Devices	All Women	All Women	All Women
Pharmacologic prophylaxis	For women at high risk of VTE Risks include personal history of VTE, presence of thrombophilia, presence of infection/ hemorrhage at the time of delivery, and comorbidities including HTN, obesity, autoimmune disease, sickle cell disease, multiple gestation, preeclampsia	For 10 d for women after nonelective cesarean delivery For 10 d for women after elective cesarean delivery with risk factors For 6 wk for women after cesarean delivery with risks for VTE	For all women after cesarean delivery without contraindications to LMWH, OR for women with risk factors

Abbreviations: HTN, hypertension; LMWH, low-molecular-weight heparin; VTE, venous thromboembolism.

protocols and checklists to guide the management of a clinical situation.[28] Even if there are several accepted treatment plans, the institutional/departmental adoption of one specific management plan, by virtue of standardization alone, improves outcomes.[29]

For example, implementing standardized protocols on labor induction significantly decreases the number of failed inductions of labor and the length of labor.[30] Standardizing the administration of oxytocin for labor augmentation reduces the rates of oxytocin needed without lengthening labor and simultaneously decreases the cesarean delivery rate.[31] Similarly, in 2013, Clark and colleagues[29] proposed an algorithm for management of a category II fetal heart tracing. Use of this algorithm allows for the clinician to comply with the standard of care. It will ultimately enhance the ability to interpret fetal heart rate tracings by decreasing provider variability and subsequently standardize clinical management.

There are 2 types of variation. Necessary clinical variation is in response to individual demographics, medical history, comorbidities, and desired outcomes. Unexplained clinical variation is not necessary and leads to increased rates of errors.[28] Some patients cannot be managed by the standard protocol. The provider should carefully consider and document the rationale for any necessary deviations from protocol. Unnecessary variations should be minimized. Unexplained and unnecessary clinical variation is the enemy of safety.[28]

IMPLEMENTATION OF NEW PROGRAMS AND PRACTICES

Despite widespread encouragement and evidence supporting the use of protocols, clinical practice guidelines are not easily accepted. At times, guidelines will have limited effect on changing physician behavior.[32] Successful implementation requires support from administration, leadership, and dedication of resources. Consistent messaging and improved coordination among nursing, physician, physician extenders, and ancillary staff are imperative. Optimal use of information technology, effective education, and ongoing evaluation of hospital culture and practice is key to successful implementation. The ability to monitor the success of the new practice is also key to continuing to move forward.[14]

The MEWC was implemented in a variety of clinical settings. Implementation experience varied somewhat between hospitals; however, some common barriers to implementation were seen among all sites[14]:

- Lack of multidisciplinary coordination and buy-in
- Inadequate education
- Clash with hospital culture and practices
- Lack of leadership support
- Misalignment with other quality or safety initiatives

Implementation of new practices is never easy, but with the right tools and personnel it can be a success. Once implemented, ongoing monitoring of outcomes from new practice guidelines is imperative for continuous quality improvement. A root cause analysis is a powerful tool to aid in this process. If there is an adverse outcome despite compliance with a given bundle, health care providers can investigate using this tool to potentially modify the guideline and prevent future problems. The Joint Commission and the Accreditation Council for Graduate Medical Education recommend routine root cause analysis (RCA) when maternal morbidity or mortality occurs, or when there is a near miss. RCA is a critical tool for learning and prevention. RCAs answer 4 questions:

1. What happened in this case?
2. What usually happens?
3. Why did this event occur?
4. What, if anything, can be done to prevent it from happening again?

The Ishikawa causal (**Fig. 2**) diagram uses a fishbone schematic to determine the contributing factors that led to the adverse effect and identify a root cause when possible. RCA is an essential part of an institution's growth toward improved patient safety and reduced morbidity and mortality.

HEALTH INFORMATION TECHNOLOGY AND PATIENT SAFETY

The Institute of Medicine states that when designed and used appropriately, health information technology (HIT) improves the performance of health professionals, reduces costs, and enhances patient safety.[33] The 2009 Health Information Technology for Economic and Clinical Health Act incentivized health care providers to make meaningful use of electronic health records (EMR),[34] and patient portals have increased access and participation in care as well as patient satisfaction.[35]

Early warning alert systems, bundles, protocols, and checklists can all be implemented and standardized through HIT. Specific EMR systems may facilitate adherence to protocols by alerting providers to abnormal clinical signs or test results and may provide decision aids for diagnostic and management plans. For example, at the authors' institution, the postoperative order set after cesarean delivery automatically includes LMWH for all patients. Therefore, providers must "opt out" of ordering LMWH if the patient does not have increased risk for VTE and they do not want the patient to receive LMWH. Although there is potential risk that a provider may not

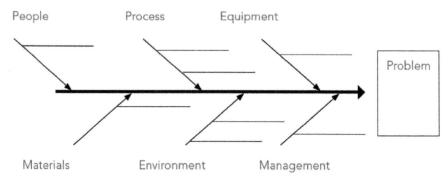

People Process Equipment

Problem

Materials Environment Management

Fig. 2. Fishbone Diagram. A common tool used in root cause analyses. (*From* Main E, Oshiro B, Chagolla B, Bingham D, Dang-Kilduff L, and Kowalewski L. Elimination of Non-medically Indicated (Elective) Deliveries Before 39 Weeks Gestational Age. (California Maternal Quality Care Collaborative Toolkit to Transform Maternity Care) Developed under contract #08-85012 with the California Department of Public Health; Maternal, Child and Adolescent Health Division; First edition published by March of Dimes, July 2010; with permission.)

opt out in a patient who does not need LMWH, the providers at Columbia University felt that far too many patients were not receiving postoperative LMWH before the implementation of this order set. The order set prompts the provider to review risk factors for VTE in every patient. Making a new practice part of an order set or protocol helps increase practice uptake and quickly makes it routine. An EMR also has the promise of collecting data and monitoring outcomes but this has not yet come to fruition in a meaningful way in most health care institutions.[14]

Incorporating HIT into patient safety programs was listed as one of the top 10 patient safety concerns in 2018 by the Emergency Care Research Institute (https://www.ecri.org). Unintended adverse events may stem from human-machine interfaces or flawed organization/system design. Excess electronic "pop-ups" designed to alert providers about potential hazards may interrupt workflow and thought processing, thereby inadvertently decreasing patient safety. Computerized physician order entry avoids illegible orders and shortens processing time of a prescription; however, the time needed to place each order has increased and the process commonly disrupts clinical workflow. Perhaps the most discouraging aspect of the EMR is that the marketplace has driven companies to develop their own proprietary systems that do not easily communicate with other EMRs. This lack of interoperability makes it nearly impossible to exchange data across and between health systems.[36]

RACIAL AND ETHNIC DISPARITIES IN MATERNAL MORBIDITY AND MORTALITY

Maternal morbidity and mortality takes a disproportionate toll on minorities in the United States. The impact of racial and ethnic disparities on maternal morbidity and mortality specifically and patient safety in general is discussed by Dr Debra Bingham and colleagues' article, "Quality Improvement Approach to Eliminate Disparities in Perinatal Morbidity and Mortality," elsewhere in this issue. Black women in the United States die at 2 to 4 times the rate of white mothers, representing one of the widest racial disparities in women's heath.[37] In 2016, the Society for Maternal Fetal Medicine noted that drivers of health disparities occur at 3 levels: (1) the patient, (2) the provider, and (3) the system.[38] ACOG and the Council on Patient Safety have published committee opinions and care bundles regarding these disparities.[39] The bundle encourages every health system to be ready to accurately obtain and document patients' self-identified race, ethnicity, and language; to recognize and provide staff-wide education on implicit bias; to respond to every clinical encounter with recognition of barriers to care; and to use reporting and systems learning to build a culture of equity.

SUMMARY

Although maternal morbidity and mortality are on the rise in the United States, this article highlights steps providers and hospitals can take to improve patient safety. The use of maternal early warning systems can help identify patients at risk. A standardized approach to major sources of morbidity and mortality, including hypertension, hemorrhage, and venous thromboembolism, will help reduce variation in care and improve outcomes. As racial disparities in maternal and neonatal outcomes are recognized and addressed, gaps in care will close. Implementation of new practices is not without challenge. Learning from each case through RCA and continuing to monitor outcomes will allow us to continue to improve patient safety.

REFERENCES

1. Callaghan WM, Creanga AA, Kuklina EV. Severe maternal morbidity among delivery and postpartum hospitalizations in the United States. Obstet Gynecol 2012; 120(5):1029–36.
2. Berg CJ, Callaghan WM, Syverson C, et al. Pregnancy-related mortality in the United States, 1998 to 2005. Obstet Gynecol 2010;116(6):1302–9.
3. D'Alton ME, Main EK, Menard MK, et al. The national partnership for maternal safety. Obstet Gynecol 2014;123(5):973–7.
4. Cantwell R, Clutton-Brock T, Cooper G, et al. Saving mothers' lives: reviewing maternal deaths to make motherhood safer: 2006-2008. The eighth report of the confidential enquiries into maternal deaths in the United Kingdom. BJOG 2011;118(Suppl 1):1–203.
5. Joint Commission on Accreditation of Healthcare Organizations, U.S.A. Preventing maternal death. Sentinel Event Alert 2010;(44):1–4.
6. Mhyre JM, D'Oria R, Hameed AB, et al. The maternal early warning criteria: a proposal from the national partnership for maternal safety. J Obstet Gynecol Neonatal Nurs 2014;43(6):771–9.
7. Duncan H, Hutchison J, Parshuram CS. The pediatric early warning system score: a severity of illness score to predict urgent medical need in hospitalized children. J Crit Care 2006;21(3):271–8.
8. Seymour CW, Liu VX, Iwashyna TJ, et al. Assessment of clinical criteria for sepsis: for the third international consensus definitions for sepsis and septic shock (Sepsis-3). JAMA 2016;315(8):762–74.
9. Lappen JR, Keene M, Lore M, et al. Existing models fail to predict sepsis in an obstetric population with intrauterine infection. Am J Obstet Gynecol 2010; 203(6):573.e1-5.
10. Hall MJ, Levant S, DeFrances CJ. Trends in inpatient hospital deaths: National Hospital Discharge Survey, 2000-2010. NCHS Data Brief 2013;(118):1–8.
11. Singh S, McGlennan A, England A, et al. A validation study of the CEMACH recommended modified early obstetric warning system (MEOWS). Anaesthesia 2012;67(1):12–8.
12. Friedman AM. Maternal early warning systems. Obstet Gynecol Clin North Am 2015;42(2):289–98.

13. Shields LE, Wiesner S, Klein C, et al. Use of maternal early warning trigger tool reduces maternal morbidity. Am J Obstet Gynecol 2016;214(4):527.e1–6.
14. Friedman AM, Campbell ML, Kline CR, et al. Implementing obstetric early warning systems. AJP Rep 2018;8(2):e79–84.
15. Smith ME, Chiovaro JC, O'Neil M, et al. Early warning system scores for clinical deterioration in hospitalized patients: a systematic review. Ann Am Thorac Soc 2014;11(9):1454–65.
16. Weiser MR, Gonen M, Usiak S, et al. Effectiveness of a multidisciplinary patient care bundle for reducing surgical-site infections. Br J Surg 2018;105(12): 1680–7.
17. Say L, Chou D, Gemmill A, et al. Global causes of maternal death: a WHO systematic analysis. Lancet Glob Health 2014;2(6):e323–33.
18. Clark SL, Hankins GD. Preventing maternal death: 10 clinical diamonds. Obstet Gynecol 2012;119(2 Pt 1):360–4.
19. Berg CJ, Harper MA, Atkinson SM, et al. Preventability of pregnancy-related deaths: results of a state-wide review. Obstet Gynecol 2005;106(6):1228–34.
20. Main EK, Goffman D, Scavone BM, et al. National partnership for maternal safety: consensus bundle on obstetric hemorrhage. Obstet Gynecol 2015;126(1): 155–62.
21. D'Alton ME, Bonanno CA, Berkowitz RL, et al. Putting the "M" back in maternal-fetal medicine. Am J Obstet Gynecol 2013;208(6):442–8.
22. Clark SL. Strategies for reducing maternal mortality. Semin Perinatol 2012;36(1): 42–7.
23. Committee on Obstetric, Practice. Committee Opinion No. 692: emergent therapy for acute-onset, severe hypertension during pregnancy and the postpartum period. Obstet Gynecol 2017;129(4):e90–5.
24. Khan KS, Wojdyla D, Say L, et al. WHO analysis of causes of maternal death: a systematic review. Lancet 2006;367(9516):1066–74.
25. ACOG Practice Bulletin No. 196: thromboembolism in pregnancy: correction. Obstet Gynecol 2018;132(4):1068.
26. Friedman AM, D'Alton ME. Venous thromboembolism bundle: risk assessment and prophylaxis for obstetric patients. Semin Perinatol 2016;40(2):87–92.
27. Booker WA, Siddiq Z, Huang Y, et al. Use of antihypertensive medications and uterotonics during delivery hospitalizations in women with asthma. Obstet Gynecol 2018;132(1):185–92.
28. Committee on Patient Safety and Quality Improvement. Committee Opinion No. 629: clinical guidelines and standardization of practice to improve outcomes. Obstet Gynecol 2015;125(4):1027–9.
29. Clark SL, Nageotte MP, Garite TJ, et al. Intrapartum management of category II fetal heart rate tracings: towards standardization of care. Am J Obstet Gynecol 2013;209(2):89–97.
30. Rhinehart-Ventura J, Eppes C, Sangi-Haghpeykar H, et al. Evaluation of outcomes after implementation of an induction-of-labor protocol. Am J Obstet Gynecol 2014;211(3):301 e1–7.
31. Clark S, Belfort M, Saade G, et al. Implementation of a conservative checklist-based protocol for oxytocin administration: maternal and newborn outcomes. Am J Obstet Gynecol 2007;197(5):480.e1-5.
32. Cabana MD, Rand CS, Powe NR, et al. Why don't physicians follow clinical practice guidelines? A framework for improvement. JAMA 1999;282(15):1458–65.

33. Committee on Patient Safety and Health Information Technology; Institute of Medicine. In Health IT and patient safety: building safer systems for better care. Washington, DC: National Academies Press; 2011.
34. Kruse CS, Bolton K, Freriks G. The effect of patient portals on quality outcomes and its implications to meaningful use: a systematic review. J Med Internet Res 2015;17(2):e44.
35. Neuner J, Fedders M, Caravella M, et al. Meaningful use and the patient portal: patient enrollment, use, and satisfaction with patient portals at a later-adopting center. Am J Med Qual 2015;30(2):105–13.
36. Committee on Patient Safety and Quality Improvement, Committee on Practice Management. Committee opinion no. 621: patient safety and health information technology. Obstet Gynecol 2015;125(1):282–3.
37. Tucker MJ, Berg CJ, Callaghan WM, et al. The Black-White disparity in pregnancy-related mortality from 5 conditions: differences in prevalence and case-fatality rates. Am J Public Health 2007;97(2):247–51.
38. Jain JA, Temming LA, D'Alton ME, et al. SMFM special report: putting the "M" back in MFM: reducing racial and ethnic disparities in maternal morbidity and mortality: a call to action. Am J Obstet Gynecol 2018;218(2):B9–17.
39. ACOG Committee Opinion No. 649: racial and ethnic disparities in obstetrics and gynecology. Obstet Gynecol 2015;126(6):e130–4.

Benefits and Pitfalls of Ultrasound in Obstetrics and Gynecology

Ray Abinader, MD, Steven L. Warsof, MD*

KEYWORDS

• Ultrasound • Obstetrics • Gynecology • Pitfalls

KEY POINTS

• Ultrasound imaging has revolutionized the practice of Ob/Gyn.
• Ultrasound can be used to determine fetal viability, gestational age, multiple gestations, morphology, growth, and fetal weight.
• Although powerful diagnostic tool, many potential sources of errors that could lead to poor outcomes.

INTRODUCTION

Ultrasonics in medicine was initially used for therapy in neurosurgery and rehabilitation medicine rather than diagnosis.[1] Its first diagnostic application came in the 1940s and eventually in Obstetrics and Gynecology (Ob/Gyn) in the 1950s.[2] With technical advances from A mode, B mode, gray scale, real time, Doppler flow analysis, color Doppler, and now to 3D and 4D imaging, this technology has given the obstetrician and gynecologist and their patient an unprecedented window into the pelvis and the fetal environment.

With ultrasound clinicians can more accurately assess fetal growth, identify multiple pregnancies and fetal and placental abnormalities, and investigate pelvic masses. Ultrasound examination is now recommended for screening all pregnant patients as well as for the diagnosis of numerous gynecologic pathologies. This imaging modality has become an integral part of routine Ob/Gyn care. It is difficult to imagine how Ob/Gyn was practiced without ultrasound.

Since ultrasound was incorporated into practice, there has been a continual evolution in training and quality. For many years, obstetricians were encouraged to purchase ultrasound machines for their office despite minimal training during their

Nothing to disclose.
Maternal Fetal Medicine, Eastern Virginia Medical School, 825 Fairfax Avenue, Norfolk, VA 23507, USA
* Corresponding author.
E-mail address: warsofsl@evms.edu

residencies, which often left them unprepared to perform quality scanning. As the years progressed, scanning became increasingly an integral part of residency training. In addition, ultrasound and radiology schools were developed to train sonographers who were certified by the American Registry for Diagnostic Sonography (ARDMS). The sonographers worked collaboratively alongside physicians in both inpatient and outpatient settings. Ultrasound availability and quality improved. By the mid-1990s routine obstetric scanning was available for almost all pregnancies. However, as equipment became more sophisticated and technical skills improved, expectations increased.

Initially tiers of scanning capabilities were established, the so-called level I, II, or III scan, but it soon became evident that there needed to be uniformity in quality and content of scanning. Through the efforts of the American Institute of Ultrasound in Medicine (AIUM), the American College of Obstetricians and Gynecologists (ACOG), the American College of Radiology, and the Society of Maternal Fetal Medicine, indications and guidelines were developed.

Despite all the potential benefits of ultrasound use in obstetrics and gynecology, there are also many potential pitfalls. Expectations from patients as to what can or should be identified have also increased. In this setting of high technology and high patient expectations, the potential for misdiagnosis and issues of patient safety are common.

This article discusses in depth the various applications for ultrasound in Ob/Gyn and the various pitfalls one can encounter; this is reviewed in an illustrative case presentation format.

OBSTETRIC ULTRASOUND EVALUATION
First Trimester

Real-time ultrasound transducers were initially designed for second-trimester scanning. First-trimester scans were not performed routinely because the uterus was still a pelvic organ and therefore was not accurately visualized through the abdomen. With advances in ultrasound transducers, including transvaginal probes with higher and variable frequencies and focal lengths, ultrasound evaluation of the first-trimester fetus and its environment became possible.[3] The first-trimester scan initially was used for confirming fetal viability, excluding ectopic pregnancies, early and more precise dating of pregnancies, and identifying the chorionicity in multiple gestations. Only recently has it also been recognized as an essential tool in screening for major fetal anomalies and aneuploidies earlier in pregnancy.

There are now published guidelines for the performance of the first-trimester ultrasound scan from the International Society of Ultrasound in Obstetrics and Gynecology (ISUOG), AIUM, and the German Society of Ultrasound in Medicine.[3] With standardization came the expectation that scans would conform to this "standard of care". Failure to perform scans at the level of the "standard of care" leads to the potential of significant safety issues. Indications for first-trimester scan aside from pregnancy evaluation include any unusual pelvic pain, bleeding, inconsistency with physical examination, or any suspicion of fetal anomaly.

Box 1 details the purposes of performing the first-trimester ultrasound examination. **Box 2** outlines the anatomic features that should be identified in the late first-trimester examination performed at 11 to 14 weeks' gestation.

Despite its utility, first-trimester screening ultrasound examination is complex and has significant limitations and pitfalls. Significant errors include incorrect dating, erroneous aneuploidy screening methodology, misdiagnosed or missed major fetal

Box 1
Purposes of the first-trimester ultrasound scan
Identification of an intrauterine pregnancy
Confirmation of fetal viability (presence of fetal heart activity)
Identification of multiple gestation with determination of fetal number and chorionicity
Assessment of gestational age
Assessment of basic fetal anatomy

anomalies, missed ectopic or heterotopic pregnancy, missed adnexal masses, missed placental or cord anomalies, missed multiple gestation, and misdiagnosis of chorionicity. The following cases elucidate how such errors could occur in clinical practice.

Case 1: The dating error
Patient presented for her first ultrasonogram during the pregnancy. Based on a confident last menstrual period (LMP), gestational age was 12 weeks (12 wga). The ultrasound scan, however, revealed a gestational age of 9 weeks based on crown-to-rump length (CRL). The estimated delivery date was not adjusted at that time. Pregnancy progressed with no complications and a repeat cesarean section was performed at 39 wga based on her dates but was 36 wga based on the first-trimester ultrasound scan. The infant was delivered uneventfully but immediately started retracting, and did not respond to resuscitative measures. Eventually he was transferred to area Newborn ICU and intubated, but developed persistent pulmonary hypertension and died after prolonged hospitalization.

In this case, the estimated due date should have been adjusted based on the early ultrasound examination and documented clearly in the medical record to prevent iatrogenic premature delivery. The fetal outcome probably would then have been very different.

Dating errors are more likely to occur the later the mother presents for prenatal care. Obstetric ultrasound scans are limited in their ability to date a pregnancy especially

Box 2
Fetal anatomy identified during the early first-trimester ultrasound scan
Head: presence, calvarium, midline falx, lateral ventricle, cerebellum
Neck: nuchal translucency area
Face: eyes, profile, and cleft
Spine: vertebrae
Chest: lung fields
Cardiac: regular rhythm and appropriately sized and symmetrical chambers
Abdomen: stomach bladder and kidneys
Extremities: 4 limbs with all bones and proper orientation
Placenta and cord: 3-vessel cord, cord insertion, and appropriate location of placenta

after 22 weeks of gestation.[4] In May 2017, ACOG published a committee opinion with current guidelines for pregnancy dating.[4] The earlier the obstetric ultrasound scan is done, the more precise the dating. Dating done prior to 14 weeks gestation should be adjusted based on the crown-to-rump (CRL) measurements if the discrepancy between gestational age based on LMP and that based on the CRL is more than 5 days at a gestational age of less than 9 weeks gestation, and if the discrepancy is more than 7 days if the gestational age is between 9 weeks and 14 weeks gestation.[4] Dating done after 14 weeks gestation should be adjusted based on the fetal biometry measurements (BPD, HC, AC, FL) with a discrepancy of more than 7, 10, 14 and 21 days used as cutoffs for redating at gestational ages of 14-16, 16-22, 22-28, and >28 weeks respectively.[4]

Case 2: The misdiagnosed/mismanaged ectopic pregnancy

A woman presented at presumed 7 weeks of gestation based on her last menstrual period. A transvaginal ultrasound scan (TVUS) showed a right adnexal complex mass and fluid in the uterus without evidence of an intrauterine gestation. A second TVUS was then performed 2 days later, which again did not show an intrauterine pregnancy. The β-human chorionic gonadotropin (β-HCG) was 917 mIU/mL. The patient was given methotrexate (MTX) to end the presumed ectopic pregnancy. Follow-up β-HCG levels on days 4 and 7 showed that her serum β-HCG level had risen to 4757 mIU/mL rather than falling in response to the MTX. The patient received a second dose of MTX. Follow-up β-HCG levels continued to increase. A repeat ultrasound scan noted the presence of a viable intrauterine pregnancy at 5 weeks of gestation. The right adnexal mass was a hemorrhagic corpus luteum cyst. Subsequent scans showed the fetus with multiple anomalies attributed to MTX exposure. The intrauterine pregnancy was terminated.

Dating adjustments based on ultrasonography should not be done after the late second trimester unless a discrepancy of more than 21 days is present. Pregnancies dated by an ultrasound scan at or beyond 22 weeks of gestation should be considered suboptimally dated[4] and fetal lung maturity should be documented before an elective delivery.

In the early first trimester, from 4 to 8 weeks of gestation, scanning can answer 3 important questions:

- Are you pregnant?
- Where is the pregnancy located?
- Is the pregnancy viable?

Vaginal bleeding and/or pelvic cramping early in the first trimester are common occurrences and may pose a difficult diagnostic challenge. The first structure visualized in a normal pregnancy is the gestational sac, which can be seen as early as 4 to 5 weeks of gestation. By 5 to 6 weeks of gestation the yolk sac should be visible and by 6 to 7 weeks, the embryo should be evident.[5] Pregnancy viability is usually defined by the presence of an embryo and identification of a fetal heartbeat at a normal rate (120–160 beats/min). Viability can usually be confirmed, using TVUS, by 7 to 8 weeks of gestation.[6]

The ability to detect pregnancy at a much earlier gestational age before all 3 questions can be accurately answered led to transitional diagnosis of pregnancy of unknown location (PUL) or pregnancy of unknown viability (PUV).[7] A definite diagnosis of intrauterine pregnancy is made on visualization of an intrauterine gestational sac containing either a yolk sac or embryo, or both. A definite diagnosis of ectopic pregnancy is made when a gestational sac containing either a yolk sac or embryo, or both, is identified outside the uterus. The temporary diagnosis of PUL applies if neither criterion is met. This diagnostic uncertainty can be resolved with time by closely monitoring the patient's signs and symptoms, serial β-HCG measurements, and ultrasound scans. Typically an intrauterine pregnancy can be identified with β-HCG of 1500 mIU/mL. This is frequently referred to as the discriminatory level, but on rare occasions an intrauterine pregnancy may not be identified until a β-HCG level of 3500 mIU/mL is reached.[8]

In case 2, solely relying on the ultrasound findings and not correlating it with the β-HCG values led to errors in diagnosis and treatment. Instead there should have been the temporary diagnosis of PUL. With patience and further evaluation, an intrauterine pregnancy would have been identified.

Second and Third Trimester

There is a growing list of indications for ultrasound scanning in the second and third trimesters (**Box 3**).[9] As indications become more numerous, so do the potential pitfalls. By understanding the limitations of obstetric ultrasound in the second and third trimester, fetal and maternal complications can be reduced.

Case 3: The Short Cervix

A 28-year-old G2 P0101 patient had a history of preterm labor with prolonged hospitalization for advanced cervical dilation 13 years previously. She eventually delivered a viable infant at 34 weeks' gestation. She presented early in this pregnancy for prenatal care with the hope of decreasing her risk of recurrent preterm labor and delivery. At 18 weeks of gestation, the ultrasound cervical length was normal at 3.4 cm. A repeat ultrasound cervical length 2 weeks later at 20 weeks of gestation reported a cervical length of 4.1 cm. At 23 weeks of gestation, the patient presented with pelvic cramping and spotting. The cervix was dilated 5 cm and there was fetal bradycardia. Given the patient's desire to have everything done to save the fetus' life, an emergency cesarean section was performed. The infant was depressed at birth and later developed cerebral palsy and severe developmental delay. Review of prior ultrasound images noted that the cervical length measured at 20 weeks of gestation was 4.1 mm, not 4.1 cm! Had the short cervical length been treated with activity restrictions, progesterone support, and emergent cerclage, the outcome might have been different.

Box 3
Elements to be identified during second-trimester and third-trimester ultrasound scans

Fetal lie, presentation, position, and number with chorionicity

Cardiac activity and heart rate

Basic fetal biometry and estimated fetal weight

Basic fetal anatomy (similar to first-trimester anatomy scan but in more detail, including cardiac outflow tracks)

Cervical length when appropriate

Placental location, with evaluation for placenta accreta and amniotic fluid assessment

Assessment of adnexa

Adapted from Abuhamad A, Chaoui R, Jeanty P, et al. Stepwise standardized approach to the basic obstetric ultrasound examination in the second and third trimester. In: Ultrasound in obstetrics and gynecology: a practical approach, 1st edition. 2014; with permission.

Cervical length assessment, usually performed in the second trimester (16–24 weeks of gestation), is an important sonographic tool to identify women at high risk of preterm delivery. With proper identification of women with a shortened cervix, the clinician can intervene to prevent, delay, or prepare for preterm birth. Despite it being the best clinical predictor of spontaneous preterm delivery, false negatives and false positives are not uncommon and underscore the importance of optimal image acquisition and measurement of the cervix. In 2011, the Perinatal Quality Foundation convened a cervix education task force, which developed consensus criteria for sonographic cervical measurements during pregnancy. This led to the development of the Cervical Length Education and Review (CLEAR) program.[10] Providers performing cervical length evaluations should be certified by the CLEAR program, which has been accepted by the American Board of Obstetrics and Gynecology for maintenance of certification of cervical length assessments.[11]

There are both anatomic and technical pitfalls that confound a cervical length assessment. Anatomic pitfalls that impede proper measurement of the cervical length include an undeveloped lower uterine segment, focal myometrial contractions, overdistended bladder, rapid and spontaneous cervical change, and cervical lesions such as polyps.[12] Technical pitfalls include incorrect vaginal probe orientation resulting in misdiagnosis of the internal os dilation, distortion of the cervix by the transducer resulting in artificial lengthening of the endocervical canal, and improper caliper placement.[13–15]

Case 3 illustrates an even more basic error: confusing "cm" and "mm" in reporting the cervical length. This report falsely reassured the provider that the cervical length was normal, thereby preventing early intervention.

Erroneous measurement of the cervical length, as illustrated in this case, can lead to catastrophic fetal morbidity and mortality with long-standing consequences for the fetus and mother. A standardized method to ensure good-quality images is essential for reproducible measurements. With the newly adopted incorporation of universal cervical length assessment in most maternal-fetal medicine centers, it is imperative that providers be wary of falsely reassuring findings arising from potential anatomic, technical, or mathematical errors.

Case 4: The Missed Fetal Anomaly

A 38-year-old G2 P0101 presented for prenatal care. She was known to have multiple pregnancy risk factors including morbid obesity with body mass index (BMI) of 62, chronic hypertension, and a history of a prior cesarean section at 35 weeks. Her estimated date of confinement (EDC) was confirmed by an ultrasound scan at 14 weeks' gestation. The patient desired as many tests as possible to ensure that the baby was "okay." Genetic and diabetic screening was normal. Her blood pressure had been well controlled without medications. Second-trimester ultrasound examinations were performed at 18, 22, and 24 weeks of gestation. All were reported as normal although all were limited by maternal body habitus. No major fetal anomalies were noted. The pregnancy progressed well until 35 weeks' gestation when she had premature rupture of membranes. She ultimately underwent a repeat cesarean section for failure to progress in labor. The live born infant was noted to have ambiguous genitalia, imperforate anus, trachea-esophageal fistula, and an absent right kidney consistent with VATER (Vertebrae, Anus, Trachea, Esophagus, and/or Renal abnormality) association. The newborn was taken to a regional perinatal center with subsequent multiple surgeries and developed cerebral palsy with severe neurologic developmental delay. The family claimed that the physician performed unsafe ultrasound evaluations. On closer scrutiny, the ultrasound practice was not AIUM accredited, the ultrasound equipment was outdated, and the sonographers were not certified Registered Diagnostic Medical Sonographers. The patient stated that she was always reassured by the scans despite the inability to see all the fetal structures required for the basic ultrasound examination. At no time was it suggested that the patient be referred to a maternal-fetal medicine practice with an accredited sonography program. The patient stated that she would have driven anywhere for a more thorough evaluation. Had she known of the fetal malformations she would have terminated the pregnancy.

Box 4
Basic fetal anatomy in the second and third trimesters of pregnancy

Head: lateral cerebral ventricles, midline falx, cavum septum pellucidum, choroid plexus, thalami, cerebellum, foramen magna, philtrum, and upper lip

Chest: 4-chamber view of the heart with orientation in the chest, right and left outflow tracts, lung fields

Abdomen: stomach with situs, bladder, kidneys, umbilical cord insertion, 3-vessel cord

Skeletal: spine seen in its entirety, all 4 limbs and their orientation

Placental: location, adnexae, and amniotic fluid level

Adapted from Abuhamad A, Chaoui R, Jeanty P, et al. Stepwise standardized approach to the basic obstetric ultrasound examination in the second and third trimester. In: Ultrasound in obstetrics and gynecology: a practical approach, 1st edition. 2014; with permission.

One of the main objectives of a second-trimester ultrasound examination is to evaluate fetal anatomy and exclude congenital defects. This fetal morphology scan is usually performed during 18 to 22 weeks of gestation. National guidelines have been established by AIUM (www.AIUM.org) and international guidelines by ISUOG (www.ISUOG.org) to optimally obtain appropriate views of numerous fetal organs to ensure normalcy. The basic fetal anatomy that should be obtained during second-trimester ultrasound examination is listed in **Box 4**.[9] Providers and sonographers performing such examinations should be properly trained and qualified. One of the greatest pitfalls of obstetric ultrasound is inadequate evaluation resulting from inadequate training, equipment, or accreditation. The failure to diagnosis either a major or minor congenital anomaly can be devastating to the family. Optimal image acquisition is essential to obtain most of the views required in the basic second-trimester ultrasound examination. To be proficient, the sonographer should have a good understanding of the physical principles of ultrasound, the basic operations of the ultrasound equipment, basic technical skills, and knowledge of the relevant anatomy. Image quality can be affected by maternal or fetal position, placental location, ultrasound machine settings, probe selection and orientation, maternal weight, amniotic fluid volume, and, most importantly, the experience of the operator.

In case 4, many of the limitations of second-trimester ultrasound examination were encountered. This case demonstrates the importance of appropriate training, equipment, knowledge, and documentation of the basic ultrasound examination in compliance with guidelines set by AIUM or ISUOG. When there are any questions about the examination, there should be no hesitation to refer the patient to a higher-level imaging center. Despite the determination of a normal fetal anatomy earlier in gestation, repeat ultrasound examinations are recommended. Many fetal malformations may not appear until later in gestation, and some abnormalities could have been missed in prior ultrasound examinations.[9] The "informal bedside" examination without documentation should be avoided whenever possible because lack of documentation and quality control may result in erroneous information.

Case 5: The Erroneous Estimated Fetal Weight

A 35-year-old woman, G1 P0 with history of gestational diabetes and a BMI of 42, presented to Labor and Delivery for induction of labor at 41 weeks of gestation. Before induction of labor, the ultrasound measurement of the estimated fetal weight (EFW) was 4250 g. The induction was then started and progressed slowly but uneventfully. After 30 hours of labor the cervix became fully dilated. After the patient pushed for 1.5 hours, the fetal head was delivered.

A shoulder dystocia was encountered. The fetus was unable to be delivered despite McRobert's maneuver and suprapubic pressure. Additional maneuvers were also unsuccessful. An emergency cesarean section was ordered, but the baby died before it could be performed. The birth weight was 4725 g. The patient claimed that she should have been offered a primary cesarean section for fetal macrosomia in a mother with gestational diabetes mellitus. Review of the ultrasound images used to estimate the fetal weight confirmed poor image acquisition, especially for the measurement of the abdominal circumference.

"Know and follow management guidelines." This is especially true for the estimation of the fetal weight whereby small measurement errors result in dramatic differences in the EFW. It is even more significant at the extremes of EFW, where accuracy is most important. These errors would adversely affect obstetric management. Providers performing and reading the ultrasound scan should obtain the optimal images complying with accepted guidelines to obtain the best estimate of the fetal weight. Sonographers performing the ultrasound scan should be mindful of the correct orientation for the ultrasound probe to measure biparietal diameter, head circumference, abdominal circumference, and femur length, and also correct caliper-placement end points. Guidelines have been established by AIUM and ISUOG and should be carefully followed.[16,17] Inability to properly see the skin edges because of fetal positioning, oligohydramnios, shadowing of fetal parts, or placental location affects all these measures. Despite these limitations that could impede proper image acquisition, expertise in scanning allows the operator to find proper planes to optimize the images.

Even with optimal ultrasound images, the EFW has innate limitations with up to 20% variability.[18] This is especially true in late gestations owing to fetal crowding. In case 5, the EFW was difficult to obtain because of maternal obesity, oligohydramnios, and fetal crowding, which led to the erroneous EFW of 4250 g, below ACOG's guideline of 4500 g to consider a cesarean section for a diabetic pregnant woman. It is therefore important to counsel any patient about the innate limitation of the ultrasound scan in estimating the fetal weight.

Case 6: The inappropriate Biophysical profile

A 27-year-old G1 P0 woman presented to the hospital at 36 1/7 weeks of gestation complaining of decreased fetal movements over the past day. The fetal monitor showed a heart rate of 125 beats/min with minimal variability, no accelerations, and no decelerations. With a nonreactive nonstress test (NST), the obstetrician ordered a biophysical profile (BPP). In the radiology department a skilled sonographer performed the BPP. The patient returned to Labor and Delivery 90 minutes later. The BPP was 2/10. The mother was placed back on the fetal monitor, which showed minimal variability and then a sudden bradycardia, unresponsive to external resuscitative measures. An emergency cesarean section was performed with delivery of a severely depressed male infant. He had a low Apgar score and an umbilical artery cord pH of 6.98. The newborn was placed on hypothermia protocol. The child survived but developed severe cerebral palsy. Concern was raised that the initial fetal heart tracing warranted immediate intervention, especially considering the length of time that the patient was in the radiology department. The sonographer reported that she could tell almost immediately that the fetus had no movements or tone but as per protocol for a BPP, observed the fetus for at least 30 minutes. In addition, after completion of the BPP there was delay in returning the mother to Labor and Delivery because the transporter was on break.

Third-trimester ultrasound evaluations can be used to assess fetal well-being and prevent fetal morbidity and mortality. Current fetal surveillance tests include the NST, contractions stress test, BPP, modified BPP, maternal perception of fetal movement, and umbilical artery Doppler velocimetry,[19] all of which have a high negative predictive value regarding the low risk of fetal acidemia. The NST only records the relationship of fetal heart rate to fetal movement. The BPP requires the performance of an NST as well as an ultrasound examination to determine fetal movements, fetal tone, and fetal breathing, and to assess amniotic fluid volume. Compared with the NST, the BPP is operator dependent, time consuming, and expensive. The false-positive rate for the BPP is high, and results should always be considered in the context of the overall clinical picture.[19] Several factors, such as maternal hypoxia, ruptured membranes, certain medications, or illicit drugs, may affect the reliability of BPP as well as other antepartum tests.[20] In case 6 there were 3 problems with the BPP. First, the patient was taken off the monitor and brought to the radiology department. Second, the sonographer watched the ultrasonogram for 30 minutes despite realizing that the fetus was in distress shortly after the scan started. The patient should have been returned immediately to Labor and Delivery with an explanation of the sonographer's concern. Third, there was a significant delay in returning the patient to Labor and Delivery even after fetal distress was recognized. All 3 of these problems represent system issues beyond the control of the individual clinician.

GYNECOLOGIC ULTRASOUND EVALUATION

Ultrasound evaluation is also critical in gynecologic diagnosis and management. Ultrasound assessment is important in the evaluation of adnexal masses, endometrium, uterine anatomy, and other pelvic structures.

Ultrasound is also the most optimal imaging modality for uterine assessment. 3D ultrasound aids in the diagnosis of uterine malformations and uterine fibroids. It is also used in the evaluation of patients with abnormal uterine bleeding or postmenopausal bleeding. In these patients, ultrasonography can be used to measure the endometrial thickness as well as the presence of polyps and submucosal, intramural, or subserosal fibroids. The use of a saline-infused sonohysterogram can further improve the diagnosis of organic endometrial anomalies such as submucosal fibroids or polyps.

Case 7: Evaluation of Adnexal Mass

A 56-year-old woman with a family history of ovarian cancer had pelvic ultrasound scans every 6 months to evaluate a persistent left ovarian cyst. Although measured correctly at each scan, there was no mention of the changing appearance of the cyst and its complex appearance with neovascularity, and the development of papillary projections and excrescences. When the patient developed significant left lower quadrant pain, exploratory surgery was performed and stage III ovarian cancer was diagnosed. In this case, failing to use ultrasonography to characterize the appearance and vascularity of a persistent ovarian cyst in a woman at high risk for ovarian cancer led to a delayed diagnosis.

Ultrasonography is critical for the assessment of adnexal masses. The structural features, size and vascularity, and their changes over time help guide clinical decisions in the management of these masses.

Case 8: Evaluation of Postmenopausal Bleeding

A 63-year-old postmenopausal woman presented with a single episode of vaginal bleeding. A pelvic ultrasound scan was performed and reported as benign. Her symptoms resolved but returned 6 months later. The patient ignored the return of occasional vaginal bleeding as she was reassured by her prior normal ultrasound evaluation. When bleeding persisted, the patient returned to her gynecologist. Dilatation and curettage diagnosed endometrial cancer. Review of the original scan revealed a significantly thickened endometrium.

Familiarity with gynecologic scanning and measurements are key to early diagnosis of malignancy. In both cases the sonographer, although fairly experienced in obstetric scanning, had only recently expanded his/her practice to include gynecologic scanning and had little experience or training in gynecologic scanning.

In case 8, if there was any uncertainty, a saline-infusion hysterosonogram, a valuable adjunct in assessing the endometrium, should have been recommended. Furthermore, the patient should have been counseled about the inherent limitations in ultrasound evaluation of the endometrium. She should have been told to immediately report any recurrence of bleeding for further evaluation.

Despite all its potential benefits, there are still many pitfalls and limitations of gynecologic ultrasound assessment. These may be related to technique, protocol, or interpretation of images, all of which could lead to errors in diagnosis. Complicating the interpretation of ultrasound images in the pelvis is the presence of many organs including the uterus, fallopian tubes, and adnexa as well as the bowels, bladder, ureter, nerves, and blood vessels. Nongynecologic pelvic structures may affect the ultrasound evaluation. For example, in the setting of dermoid cysts a loop of bowel can be mistaken for a dermoid plug, leading to erroneous diagnosis and unnecessary surgery. Peristalsis, not visible on a still image, is critical in distinguishing loops of bowel from a dermoid cyst. Presence or absence of peristalsis must therefore be communicated by the sonographer to the physician.

Ultrasound images of fibroids can also be misinterpreted. An exophytic subserosal fibroid on an ultrasonogram might be diagnosed as a solid adnexal mass leading to unnecessary surgery. When fibroids undergo degeneration, they may also develop rim-enhancing calcifications and may be confused with adnexal disorder.

By standardizing the scanning process and following accepted guidelines, errors related to technique may be minimized. Complying with the certification criteria for equipment and personnel will further reduce errors and improve safety.

SUMMARY

Given the rapid advances in knowledge and equipment in ultrasonography, it is imperative for practitioners performing and interpreting ultrasound examinations to stay current regarding guidelines, protocols, and policies to maintain a safe practice.

With the growing value of ultrasound in modern obstetrics and gynecology, integration of this tool in everyday practice is essential. Knowing when to refer a patient to a specialist for a more comprehensive ultrasound evaluation is often a difficult decision. Appropriate referral may help prevent errors from misdiagnosis of an ultrasound scan. Irrespective of the level of ultrasound evaluation, it is important to provide and maintain the best equipment possible. Certification of personnel and compliance with protocols is also important. Ultrasound evaluations, especially in cases of misdiagnosis, should undergo periodic, retrospective reviews as part of a continuous quality improvement program. All images, loop videos, and reports should be properly archived.

The ultrasound examination is a valuable tool. By knowing the limitations and pitfalls of ultrasound, providers can more appropriately manage and counsel patients.

REFERENCES

1. Miller DL, Smith NB, Bailey MR, et al. Overview of therapeutic ultrasound applications and safety considerations. J Ultrasound Med 2012;31(4):623–34.
2. Carovac A, Smajlovic F, Junuzovic D. Application of ultrasound in medicine. Acta Inform Med 2011;19(3):168–71.
3. Abuhamad A. Guidelines to fetal imaging in the first trimester. In: Abuhamad A, Chaoui R, editors. First trimester ultrasound diagnosis of fetal abnormalities. Philadelphia: Wolter Kluwer; 2018. p. 3–8.
4. ACOG's Committee on Obstetric Practice. Methods for estimating the due date. ACOG Committee Opinion No: 700. Obstet Gynecol 2017;129(5):e150–4.
5. Cohen L. Diagnostic ultrasound in the first trimester of pregnancy. In: Global library of women's medicine. 2008. https://doi.org/10.3843/GLOWM.10094 (ISSN: 1756-2228).
6. Rodgers S, Chang C, DeBardeleben J, et al. Normal and abnormal US findings in early first- trimester pregnancy: review of the society of radiologists in ultrasound 2012 consensus panel recommendations. Radiographics 2015;35:2135–48.
7. Myer E, Arrington J, Warsof S. Pregnancy of unknown viability. In: Stadtmauer L, Tur-Kaspa I, editors. Ultrasound imaging in reproductive medicine. New York: Springer Science and Business Media; 2014. p. 315–27.
8. Committee on Practice Bulletins—Gynecology. Tubal ectopic pregnancy. Practice Bulletin 193. Obstet Gynecol 2017;131(2):e65–77.
9. Abuhamad A, Chaoui R, Jeanty P, et al. Ultrasound in obstetrics and gynecology: a practical approach 2014. p. 66–121.
10. Cervical length education and review. Available at: https://clear.perinatalquality.org/. Accessed September 3, 2018.
11. Society for Maternal-Fetal Medicine (SMFM), McIntosh J, Feltovich H, Berghella V, et al. The role of routine cervical length screening in selected high- and low-risk women for preterm birth prevention. Am J Obstet Gynecol 2016;215(3):B2–7.
12. Yost NP, Bloom SL, Twickler DM, et al. Pitfalls in ultrasonic cervical length measurement for predicting preterm birth. Obstet Gynecol 1999;93(4):510–6.
13. Karis JP, Hertzberg BS, Bowie JD. Sonographic diagnosis of premature cervical dilatation: potential pitfall due to lower uterine segment contractions. J Ultrasound Med 1991;10:83–7.
14. Harris RD, Barth RA. Sonography of the gravid uterus and placenta: current concepts. AJR Am J Roentgenol 1993;160:455–65.
15. Parulekar SG, Kiwi R. Dynamic incompetent cervix uteri. J Ultrasound Med 1988; 7:481–5.
16. The American Institute of Ultrasound in Medicine. AIUM practice parameter for the performance of obstetric ultrasound examinations. AIUM; 2013. Laurel (MD).
17. The International Society of Ultrasound in Obstetrics and Gynecology. Practice guidelines for performance of the routine mid-trimester fetal ultrasound scan. Ultrasound Obstet Gynecol 2011;37(1):116–26.

18. Committee on Practice Bulletins—Obstetrics and the American Institute of Ultrasound in Medicine. Ultrasound in pregnancy. Practice Bulletin No: 175. Obstet Gynecol 2016;128(6):e241–56.
19. ACOG's Committee on Practice Bulletins. Antepartum fetal surveillance. Practice Bulletin 145. Obstet Gynecol 2014;124(1):182–92.
20. Walsh M. The biophysical profile. Global library of women's medicine 2008. https://doi.org/10.3843/GLOWM.10209 (ISSN: 1756-2228).

Patient Safety in Outpatient Procedures

Mark S. DeFrancesco, MD, MBA[a,b,c,*]

KEYWORDS

- Accreditation • Ambulatory surgery • Certification • Patient safety
- Office procedures • ASC • Ambulatory Surgery Center

KEY POINTS

- Over the past 4 decades, there has been a sea-change with many surgical procedures transitioning to ambulatory settings.
- There are multiple reasons for this transition, with benefits and drivers related to payers, providers, and patients.
- There are variations in risk profiles that seem to be dependent on site of service.
- The explosion in the number of ambulatory facilities sparked a parallel increase in the interest in accreditation and quality assurance.
- The regulatory role of specialty societies and government agencies has also expanded.

INTRODUCTION

When an otherwise healthy woman needed to undergo a procedure like a dilation and curettage for abnormal uterine bleeding as recently as the 1970s, she was required to be admitted to the hospital the day before her surgery. Then she underwent various tests, as well as the time-honored custom of completely shaving the hair in her pubic area. The latter was performed routinely, despite the lack of any evidence that doing so decreased infection or had any beneficial effect.

Usually a medical student or a resident performed an "admission history and physical" and checked laboratory results to be sure the patient was ready for surgery. Following the procedure, it was routine for the patient to stay overnight and then to be discharged home the following morning. About 40 years ago, a very minor procedure required almost 3 days out of a woman's life, 2 nights in the hospital, and a pubic shave that was otherwise neither wanted nor needed.

Today, not only "minor" cases like dilation and curettages, hysteroscopies, and tubal ligations, but major cases like hysterectomies, are performed routinely on an

Disclosure: No conflicts of interest to disclose.
[a] Department of Obstetrics and Gynecology, University of Connecticut, Storrs, CT, USA; [b] Accreditation Association for Hospitals and Health Systems (AAHHS); [c] Women's Health Connecticut
* 60 Westwood Avenue, Suite 200, Waterbury, CT 06708.
E-mail address: mdefrancesco@womenshealthct.com

Obstet Gynecol Clin N Am 46 (2019) 379–387
https://doi.org/10.1016/j.ogc.2019.01.012
0889-8545/19/© 2019 Elsevier Inc. All rights reserved.

obgyn.theclinics.com

outpatient basis. The patient is admitted to the facility an hour or so before the scheduled procedure. Pre-operative testing has already been done before admission. Because of advances in anesthesia, as well as in surgical instrumentation and techniques, many patients have major surgery performed via very tiny incisions, are given shorter-acting anesthetics and more efficient pain medications. All this allows patients to undergo even major surgery and be discharged in less than 24 hours.

In the late 1970s to the 1980s, there was a burgeoning of Ambulatory Surgery Centers (ASCs) that has accommodated the increased demand for outpatient care. In addition, since approximately 2000, there has been a further shift of many procedures from ASCs to the physician office setting. This shift was an inevitable next step in the evolution of surgical care. It also further reduced costs and sparked intensified focus on patient safety in the office setting.

In this article, the author will discuss the magnitude of the transition to more ambulatory settings and many of the drivers of this shift. Payers and providers significantly benefited from this evolution, and patients also were potential beneficiaries, especially, and only if, outcomes were as positive and as safe as they were in the hospital setting. The author will therefore also explore the safety concerns raised by this shift to the office setting.

In addition, the author will briefly trace the history of ambulatory accreditation and the role that specialty societies and governmental regulations have played in assuring safe, high-quality care in the ambulatory setting.

SEA-CHANGE IN THE SITE OF SERVICE

The most recent data available (updated in February 2018) compare the volume of ambulatory surgery as a percent of all surgeries performed in 2014 to the percent in 1994. This report demonstrated an almost 16% increase in surgeries performed in the ambulatory setting over this time span.[1] These data do not include procedures performed in physician offices, a number much more difficult to ascertain. If these were included the magnitude of the shift would be even greater.

Despite that deficit, we do know that the percentage of total outpatient encounters that take place in physician offices has increased from 82.4% in 2008, to almost 89%.[2,3] It was reported in 2007 that the number of procedures performed electively in ambulatory facilities essentially doubled to about 10 million cases.[4]

Urman and colleagues[5] in 2012 estimated that approximately 10% to 12% of ambulatory procedures were being performed in physician offices, and raised the question of "practice drift" and whether the office was becoming the "Wild West of health care," because of the lack of significant regulatory oversight of most physician offices.

REASONS FOR THE OUTPATIENT SURGERY SHIFT

The accelerating movement of surgical cases from the hospital to the ambulatory setting is a classic example of aligned incentives effecting change. All the stakeholders—patients, providers and payers—potentially benefited from the move.

First of all, but potentially least certainly a beneficiary, is the patient. As mentioned previously, the only way the patient truly benefits from the performance of her surgery or procedure in the ASC, or in the office setting especially, is if her safety and outcome are equivalent or superior to the hospital setting.

If that indeed is the case, most patients would prefer, and likely benefit from, the relative informality and warmth of a lower acuity facility. This is particularly true in the familiarity of the patient's own physician's office setting. In addition, many if not most payers require smaller or no co-pays in the ambulatory setting, another benefit to the patient.

However, this "assumption of safety" must be valid and credible. Some data suggest that procedures performed in the office setting are associated with higher adverse event rates than those in ASCs. We will discuss this in more detail in the next section. If we assume that all sites of service lead to equally good outcomes, then the patient is well-served by the movement of her surgery into less-expensive ASCs and offices.

There are potential benefits to the provider, the surgeon. Most physicians are very busy clinically and performing more procedures in the same location where they see patients is more efficient than leaving the office to go to the operating room (or even to the ASC) to perform 1 or more cases. At times cases are delayed and time is wasted. This happens less in the office setting. Physicians have more control over time, workflow, and activities in their own offices.

The payer contributes to the provider's incentive to work in ambulatory settings. Many payers use a "site of service differential" (see later discussion) that reimburses the surgeon at a higher rate if the procedure is done as an outpatient, particularly in the office setting.

Finally, payers also benefit. Why would they pay significantly more to the provider for operating in the office, as opposed to the hospital, or even an ASC? The payer typically pays lower total costs for surgery in an ASC than in a hospital, but in a physician office it would save substantially more as there are no facility fees to cover.

Many payers developed "shared savings" strategies with provider groups to encourage the shift of cases to the office setting. There are often facility fees and hospital-related charges that are lower or non-existent in ASCs and physician offices. Therefore many payers offer a site of service differential whereby the professional fee they pay the physician is significantly increased if the procedure is done in a less-expensive venue. Some of this enhanced payment is meant to recognize some increase in physician office expenses (staffing and supplies for instance) related to doing certain cases in the office, but, beyond that increment, typically a "bonus" of sorts is usually included.[6–8]

Ultimately, everyone benefits if, in fact, procedures can be pushed to the lowest acuity setting possible, but only if it is consistent with patient safety and high-quality outcomes.

PATIENT SAFETY/OUTCOMES

Several studies raised concerns about how varying the site of service affects adverse event profiles. Of note is a study from 2000 to 2002 demonstrating a significant difference (more than 10-fold increase) between adverse events and deaths in the office setting as opposed to ASCs.[9]

A more recent analysis still demonstrates a small but statistically significant difference between outcomes in physician offices versus ASCs. In this study, risk-adjusted 7- and 30-day hospital admission rates were analyzed. For women's health-related procedures, there was almost double the admission rate for office patients compared with ASC patients.[10] Clearly, additional studies are needed to resolve this concern.

Site of service most likely contributes heavily to this difference, possibly more than does the operator's credentials, experience, and training. The variables that might affect higher rates of adverse events in the office setting may be location dependent.

Why would a surgeon who presumably is performing certain procedures in a hospital or ASC without significant adverse events suddenly have a significantly increased incidence of adverse events in the office? Lack of strict adherence to accreditation-level standards in the physician office, for example, as well as much lower resource availability in terms of both staffing and equipment, might contribute to this disparity. This makes a strong case for addressing patient safety in the office setting.

However, there are other studies that fail to find any real difference in site of service outcomes. These are admittedly few and more research is needed to be more definitive about this question.[11]

At this point, there may exist safety and outcome disparities when comparing hospital and ambulatory settings. In the early years of ASC development much attention was focused on quality and safety. The early founders of ASCs originally came from hospital settings, and were aware that they needed to provide an environment that would assure the patient of an equally safe outcome. For that reason, ASCs from the earliest days adopted standards and monitored quality.

In transitioning to the office setting, however, "new wine" was being poured into "old skins." Procedures and surgeries were being moved from the formally organized environment of the hospital or ASC to the more informal and less "organized" office setting. We will first focus on ASCs, as well as accreditation and regulatory issues, after which we will look at office-based surgery and related issues and resources.

AMBULATORY SURGERY CENTER EXPLOSION

Before 1980, very few people would have predicted the incredible expansion of the ambulatory market, particularly with respect to ASCs. The first ASC was opened in Phoenix, Arizona, in 1970 by 2 surgeons looking for more autonomy, control over the schedule, better access to operating rooms and equipment, and cost-effectiveness.[12] It took a while for the concept to catch on, but by 1980, there were several hundred ASCs in operation.

In the 1980s, Medicare recognized ASCs, and by 1988 there were about 1000 ASCs.[12] Growth accelerated after the mid-1980s as many private payers in the nascent managed care era also encouraged surgeries in outpatient settings as a cost-controlling strategy. At the same time many hospitals developed joint ventures with physicians to create local ASCs. This allowed hospitals to maintain a share of the market that they were otherwise losing as surgical cases shifted to independently owned ambulatory venues. Today there are close to 6000 ambulatory surgery facilities in the United States.

Not surprisingly, as the number of ASCs grew, so too did the accreditation market. For a variety of reasons, ambulatory standards and accreditation organizations flourished over the past 30 years in response to the ASC explosion.

RISE OF ACCREDITATION ORGANIZATIONS

In the early 1970s the American Medical Association approved the concept of outpatient surgery, and anesthesia societies created initial guidelines for safety. In the late 1970s several organizations developed accreditation standards. The Accreditation Association for Ambulatory Health Care (AAAHC), became a major player in the world of ASC accreditation. It was formed in 1979 in recognition of the growing interest in ambulatory facilities, particularly free-standing surgery centers, and the relative lack of interest from what is now the Joint Commission. The Joint Commission is a major hospital-focused accreditation agency founded in 1951. It is reputed that the early pioneers who formed the AAAHC were members of the Joint Commission who were frustrated with the latter's refusal to include ambulatory facilities in its portfolio (personal informal communications with former AAAHC Board members, 2000).

Another major accreditor of ASCs is the Healthcare Facilities Accreditation Program, which was created in 1943. Unlike the Joint Commission, it readily diversified and began accrediting ambulatory facilities when their numbers increased. Though it was founded by the American Osteopathic Association to accredit osteopathic facilities, it quickly expanded its boundaries and accredits in various health care spaces, now including ambulatory.

The Healthcare Facilities Accreditation Program was acquired by the Accreditation Association for Hospitals and Health Systems (AAHHS) in 2015. The AAHHS had originated as a sister organization to the AAAHC, but separated from that group when the AAAHC opted to not enter the hospital space (personal observations and commentary of author).

Initially ambulatory surgical accreditation was purely voluntary. Only some facilities opted in. However, as early ASCs began to compete with new ones and local hospital "same day surgery" programs, accreditation became a recognized differentiator in the market place. Therefore, more facilities began to seek accredited status.

Over the next decade, accreditation became essentially mandatory. Most payers, including Medicare, began to require accreditation for reimbursement. Some states now also require even otherwise-unregulated physician offices doing procedures and using certain levels of anesthesia to be accredited. There is still wide variation in how various jurisdictions approach licensing and/or accreditation for office-based surgery, ranging from total non-regulation to full accreditation.[13]

ORIGIN OF STANDARDS

The main goal of the accreditation process is to improve the quality of care. The development of "standards" long pre-dated the establishment of accreditation agencies. The Joint Commission for example, was created in 1951 by the American College of Surgeons, the American Hospital Association, the American College of Physicians, the American Medical Association, and the Canadian Medical Association. However, surgical standards were created in 1917 to 1918 by the American College of Surgeons and were published as "Minimum Standard for Hospitals." Periodic on-site inspections of hospitals by the American College of Surgeons began at that time. These "minimum standards" were further refined and published in 1926 as an 18-page book of standards for hospitals.[14]

Today, accreditation agencies create and maintain standards for inpatient *and* outpatient facilities. The main driver for accreditation within the ambulatory setting was to help ensure that the quality of care would be comparable with accredited hospitals.

There are no accrediting agencies specifically dedicated to the office setting. A physician's office may voluntarily seek accreditation as an ambulatory site, however, but costs can be prohibitive. Few practices have the infrastructure and bandwidth required to support ongoing quality assurance programs and related quality management functions.

THE OFFICE SETTING

The Institute of Medicine's landmark publication, *To Err is Human*, had tremendous impact on formalizing a systematic response to the systematic problem of patient safety.[15] Hospitals and ASCs have used formal quality improvement activities to enhance safety and improve outcomes.[16]

However, as more procedures began moving to the office setting, and some studies demonstrated possible quality concerns related to site of service, the need for translating safety advances in inpatient and ASC environments to the office became apparent.

In 2010 the American College of Obstetricians and Gynecologists (ACOG) published its "Executive Summary of the American College of Obstetricians and Gynecologists Presidential Task Force on Patient Safety in the Office Setting."[16] This important work suggested ways to formalize procedural safety and quality in the office setting. For instance, it defined 3 levels of office procedures by level of anesthesia:

Level I: local anesthesia with minimal pre-operative oral anxiolytic medication
Level II: moderate sedation
Level III: deep sedation or general anesthesia[16]

Level III procedures require more safeguards, in both equipment and personnel, compared with level I procedures. It also encouraged the establishment of a "culture of safety," the designation of a Medical Director, the use of checklists, and generally offered strategies for formalizing safety and quality in the office.[16]

From that seminal work, 2 specific programs were developed for ACOG members, the Outpatient Safety Assessment (OPSA) and Safety Certification in Outpatient Excellence (SCOPE). Since that time, the American College of Surgeons[17] and the American Academy of Family Physicians[18] also developed policies and/or guidelines addressing this important area for their members.

EVOLUTION OF THE OUTPATIENT SAFETY ASSESSMENT AND THE SAFETY CERTIFICATION IN OUTPATIENT EXCELLENCE

The ACOG developed the OPSA tool available on its Web site. Using this tool, ACOG members could answer specific questions and evaluate their own practices vis-à-vis recommended safety practices and guidelines. A partial list of recommendations included the following:

1. Designation of a Medical Director in the practice (office) setting
2. Periodic evaluation of staff, tracking of adverse events
3. Ensuring that all laboratory and test results were communicated to patients
4. Follow-up on referrals of patients to outside specialists
5. Proper maintenance of surgical equipment and emergency packs
6. Mock safety drills

It was an opportunity to get physicians thinking about and formalizing office safety. The problem has been sustainability of this initiative.

One year after the OPSA was available online, the ACOG began to expand this concept. Recognizing that full accreditation was beyond the reach of many practices, the ACOG developed a certification program known as SCOPE. This program was intended to make certification available and affordable to most practices.

It took the elements in the OPSA program and expanded them to cover each of the following areas:

1. Office Management and Administration
2. Documentation and Reporting, Medication Safety
3. Office-Based Surgical Procedures and Equipment[19]

The SCOPE application inquires about each of these areas. The applicant completes the questionnaire online and uploads any appropriate files, such as office policies and minutes of staff meetings or mock drills.

The ACOG SCOPE staff reviews the submissions and determines if additional information is needed. If no further information is needed, they will assess the information and provide feedback to the applicant. Feedback can range from advice that they are not ready for certification owing to key deficiencies, or that all standards are generally met and they will likely be certified.

Initially every site required an on-site reviewer team to verify the information, and, if needed, offer consultative advice to help with weaker areas. However, in an effort to make the process more affordable for practices, the program was streamlined in 2016. It tried to eliminate some of the more onerous elements not directly related to patient safety and to make the site visit a possible but not definite requirement.[20]

So far, there are over 100 SCOPE-certified sites. Though the uptake is disappointing, it is understandable, given the economic limitations of many practices and the challenges of deploying the necessary infrastructure.

SCOPE might possibly evolve into an online program that would educate all ACOG members about developing and implementing safety standards in their office practices. This program would disseminate information but most likely not award certification.

FUTURE TRENDS FOR OUTPATIENT SURGERY

There are many drivers in health care today, stimulated by the need to meet the "triple aim" of better care, better cost control, and better patient experiences. Many would add a fourth aim: provider well-being. ASCs have been concerned about provider satisfaction and resilience for many years, and generally have a better relationship with members of its surgical staff than do many hospitals.[21]

Almost 90% of ASCs are wholly or partly owned by physicians. Many prefer to do their work in the ambulatory setting, as they enjoy increased control over the schedule and encounter less bureaucracy when requesting needed equipment and supplies. ASCs argue that they provide more autonomy for physicians, and surgeons seem to agree.[22]

Looking back over the past 40 years, predictions about the next 5 to 10 years regarding ASC and outpatient surgery are likely:

1. An accelerating shift of cases to the outpatient setting.
2. A 2% drop in inpatient discharges.
3. An 11% increase in outpatient surgery over the next 5 years.
4. A 15% increase in overall outpatient volumes.
5. Inpatient gynecology will drop 28%.
6. Hysterectomies will be more routinely performed in outpatient setting.
7. Due to increased adherence to obstetric guidelines and pressure from payers, overall cesarean delivery rate will drop to 26%.[23,24]

The Advisory Board follows and reports on trends. They report that health systems and non-provider organizations (such as insurance companies and "equity partners" that invest significant capital in large group practices and health care facilities) have an increased interest in ASCs that are becoming more important as cost-savers as health care transitions more from traditional "fee for service" payment systems to what is called a "value-based system."[25] This value model incentivizes providers to be more efficient while also focusing on cost and quality. Rather than traditional fee for service, a value-based system seeks alternate payment models such as capitation and "risk sharing" with providers.

SUMMARY

Since the opening of the first ASC in 1970, there has been a continuous and accelerating movement to outpatient venues, first for relatively minor surgery, and more recently for complex operations never imagined to be performed outside a hospital operating room.

This progression has been incremental. The first quantum leap was from the hospital to the ASC. This movement was initially hesitant, until the concept was proven. The true catalyst for growth, however, seems to be the recognition of outpatient facilities by Medicare and private payers.

The near-contemporaneous increase of accreditation organizations and the application of standards were found to assure the safety and quality of most accredited centers. This, then, led many states and many payers to require accreditation for licensure and payment. That requirement ultimately led to a rapid increase in the number of accredited facilities nationally.

The second significant shift was from the ambulatory surgical facility to the office. At present, with the exception of the states that require accreditation for offices that perform office-based surgery with certain levels of anesthesia (usually "moderate sedation" or deeper), there are still many jurisdictions whereby there is no regulation of in-office surgical procedures.

The ACOG, the American College of Surgeons, the American Academy of Family Physicians, and the American Society of Anesthesiologists have all created guidelines to help their members safely perform in-office surgery. Professional societies notwithstanding, there are no specific requirements in any states, other than those related to levels of anesthesia in some, to monitor compliance with these standards. Perhaps the SCOPE program can be modified to make it more accessible to all members. There is little question that the future of health care involves decentralization, at least with respect to surgical procedures. The move from the hospital to the ASC is continuing, and progressing to the physician's office for many procedures.

It is our challenge to ensure that patients are not put at risk as this trend continues.

REFERENCES

1. Available at: https://hcup-us.ahrq.gov/reports/statbriefs/sb223-Ambulatory-Inpatient-Surgeries-2014.jsp Accessed September 22, 2018.
2. Stumpf PG. Practical solutions to improve safety in the obstetrics/gynecology office setting and in the operating room. Obstet Gynecol Clin North Am 2008;35:19–35.
3. Available at: https://www.cdc.gov/nchs/fastats/physician-visits.htm Accessed September 20, 2018.
4. Shapiro FE, editor. Manual of office-based anesthesia procedures. Philadelphia: Lippincott, Williams & Wilkins; 2007.
5. Urman RD, Punwani N, Shapiro FE. Office-based surgical and medical procedures: educational gaps. Ochsner J 2012;12(4):383–8.
6. Available at: https://www.uhcprovider.com/content/dam/provider/docs/public/policies/oxford/site-of-service-differential-ohp.pdf Accessed September 12, 2018.
7. Available at: https://www.oxhp.com/secure/policy/site_of_service_differential.pdf Accessed September 12, 2018.
8. Available at: https://www.horizonblue.com/providers/policies-procedures/policies/reimbursement-policies-guidelines/site-of-service-differential Accessed September 12, 2018.
9. Vila H Jr, Soto R, Cantor AB, et al. Comparative outcomes analysis of procedures performed in Physician Offices and Ambulatory Surgery Centers. Arch Surg 2003;138(9):991–5.
10. Ohsfeldt RL, Li P, Schneider JE, et al. Outcomes of surgeries performed in physician offices compared with Ambulatory Surgery Centers and Hospital Outpatient Departments in Florida. Health Serv Insights 2017;10. 1178632917701025.

11. Berglas NF, Battistelli MF, Nicholson WK, et al. The effect of facility characteristics on patient safety, patient experience, and service availability for procedures in non-hospital-affiliated outpatient settings: a systematic review. PLoS One 2018; 13(1):e0190975. Available at: https://doi.org/10.1371/journal.pone.0190975. Accessed September 23, 2018.

12. Available at: https://www.ascassociation.org/advancingsurgicalcare/asc/historyofascs Accessed September 1, 2018.

13. Available at: http://www.physicianspractice.com/law-malpractice/what-you-need-know-about-office-based-surgery-laws Accessed September 24, 2018.

14. Available at: https://www.jointcommission.org/assets/1/6/TJC_history_timeline_through_2017.pdf Accessed September 18, 2018.

15. Kohn LT, Corrigan J, Donaldson MS. To err is human: building a safer health system. Washington, DC: National Academy Press; 2000.

16. Erickson T, Kirkpatrick D, DeFrancesco MS, et al. Executive summary of the American College of Obstetricians and Gynecologists presidential task force on patient safety in the office setting: reinvigorating safety in office-based gynecologic surgery. Obstet Gynecol 2010;115:147–51.

17. Available at: https://www.facs.org/education/patient-education/patient-safety/office-based-surgery Accessed October 5, 2018.

18. Available at: https://www.aafp.org/about/policies/all/surgery.html Accessed October 5, 2018.

19. Available at: https://www.scopeforwomenshealth.org/applying-for-scope Accessed September 20, 2018.

20. Available at: https://www.acog.org/About-ACOG/ACOG-Departments/ACOG-Rounds/April-2016/ACOG-Streamlines-SCOPE-Office-Safety-Certification-Program-Reduces-Fees Accessed September 18, 2018.

21. Available at: https://books.google.com/books?id=_NsIDwAAQBAJ&pg=PA362&lpg=PA362&dq=the+quadruple+aim+and+ASCs&source=bl&ots=DBvhpM4nCx&sig=LxrF2ddftkatlfscw7TcIQ66PRc&hl=en&sa=X&ved=2ahUKEwjCx9a7tNTdAhUQON8KHfwnD24Q6AEwCnoECAEQAQ#v=onepage&q=the%20quadruple%20aim%20and%20ASCs&f=false Accessed September 18, 2018.

22. Available at: https://www.ascassociation.org/HigherLogic/System/DownloadDocumentFile.ashx?DocumentFileKey=2e3fb5b2-0332-4af2-9537-86b8ba077a38&forceDialog=0 Accessed September 18, 2018.

23. Available at: https://www.beckersasc.com/asc-turnarounds-ideas-to-improve-performance/10-key-trends-for-ascs-and-outpatient-surgery-in-the-next-10-years.html?tmpl=component&print=1 Accessed September 20, 2018.

24. Available at: https://www.sg2.com/health-care-intelligence-blog/2017/05/sg2-2017-impact-change-forecast-finding-growth/ Accessed September 20, 2018.

25. Available at: https://www.advisory.com/research/market-innovation-center/the-growth-channel/2018/02/2018-growth-predictions Accessed September 20, 2018.

Safety in Minimally Invasive Surgery

Esther S. Han, MD, MPH[a], Arnold P. Advincula, MD[b],*

KEYWORDS

- Post-operative neuropathy • Trocar injury • Patient optimization • Safety
- Minimally invasive surgery

KEY POINTS

- Despite the many advantages of minimally invasive surgery, there are inherent risks associated with laparoscopy.
- Critical to ensuring patient safety is the need for a properly indicated procedure in the right patient performed by the appropriate surgeon.
- Prevention of post-operative neuropathy requires optimized patient positioning for surgical access without compromise to key anatomic structures.
- Safe peritoneal access necessitates an understanding of and comfort with multiple entry techniques.

Case summary

JD is a 45-year-old woman G2 P2 with a long-standing history of symptomatic uterine fibroids manifested predominantly as abnormal uterine bleeding and bulk symptoms with urinary frequency. She has failed attempts at conservative management with hormonal pharmacotherapy and an abdominal myomectomy in the remote past. Because she has completed childbearing, she now desires definitive surgical management and would like to avoid a laparotomy. A recent office endometrial biopsy was benign and the rest of her health maintenance is up to date.

Her past medical history is notable for asthma, type II diabetes, obesity, and anemia (attributable to her heavy menstrual bleeding). Her past surgical history is significant for 2 previous cesarean deliveries and the aforementioned abdominal myomectomy. On physical examination her body mass index was 30 kg/m². Her abdomen was soft and non-tender, with a palpably enlarged uterus and notable Pfannenstiel scar. The pelvic examination confirmed a 16-week size fibroid uterus with limited mobility and lack of descent. She exhibited poor access for a vaginal hysterectomy; however, she is a candidate for a conventional total laparoscopic hysterectomy with bilateral salpingectomy.

Disclosures: The authors have nothing to disclose.
[a] Division of Gynecologic Specialty Surgery, Department of Obstetrics and Gynecology, Columbia University Medical Center, New York-Presbyterian Hospital, 622 West 168th Street, PH 16, Room 139, New York, NY 10032, USA; [b] Department of Obstetrics and Gynecology, Sloane Hospital for Women, Mary & Michael Jaharis Simulation Center, Columbia University Medical Center, New York-Presbyterian Hospital, 622 West 168th Street, PH 16, Room 139, New York, NY 10032, USA
* Corresponding author.
E-mail address: aa3530@cumc.columbia.edu

Obstet Gynecol Clin N Am 46 (2019) 389–398
https://doi.org/10.1016/j.ogc.2019.01.013
0889-8545/19/© 2019 Elsevier Inc. All rights reserved.

INTRODUCTION

Every day, a countless number of patients undergo surgeries such as hysterectomy, which are performed in a minimally invasive fashion. To the busy and skilled gynecologic surgeon, the case just presented may seem routine; however, numerous safety issues are traversed in the process of completing such a surgery. It is clear that minimally invasive surgery (MIS) has numerous benefits including shorter length of hospital stay, faster return to normal activity, reduced rate of surgical site infections, less postoperative pain, less blood loss, and reduced incidence of venous thromboembolus, sepsis, and post-operative ileus.[1-4] Minimally invasive surgery can be associated with longer operative times and longer operating room (OR) times. Minimally invasive surgery has also been independently associated with increased 30-day complications after laparoscopic and robotic hysterectomies for benign indications.[5] Despite this, MIS has been shown to decrease overall complications when compared with open surgery for hysterectomies for both benign and malignant indications.[6,7] This is especially true for those women with higher body mass index (BMI), which is independently associated with significantly higher rates of venous thromboembolus and wound infection in women who had laparotomy but not in women who had MIS.[7]

Although uterine weight has been found to be an independent risk factor for posthysterectomy complications, open procedures still demonstrate significantly higher complication rates when compared with laparoscopic procedures regardless of uterine size.[4] Based on the well-documented advantages over abdominal hysterectomy, the American College of Obstetricians and Gynecologists recommends that minimally invasive approaches (vaginal or laparoscopic, including robot-assisted), should be performed, whenever feasible.[8] However, MIS has its own particular risks at the outset of the case that are associated with the mechanics of the procedures themselves, the necessary patient positioning, including steep Trendelenburg, and the need for peritoneal access. In this review, the authors focus specifically on the risks encountered with the start of a laparoscopic surgery and the ways to prevent or mitigate them.

PROCEDURE SELECTION: SHOULD A LAPAROSCOPIC APPROACH BE OFFERED?

A properly indicated procedure for the correct patient, performed by the appropriate surgeon is paramount to ensuring patient safety. In other words: right indication, right procedure, right patient, and right surgeon. The benefits of MIS must be balanced by the particular risks involved with insufflation and Trendelenburg positioning. A patient's overall health status including her comorbidities, BMI and body habitus must be carefully considered to ensure that she can tolerate the procedure and that the procedure can be safely and efficiently performed. The patient's surgical history and risk of adhesive disease, particularly when considering abdominal entry for laparoscopic trocars, should be carefully considered. Finally, the patient's pathology—size, shape, and mobility of an enlarged fibroid uterus or adnexal mass, extent of adhesive disease, and so forth—must all be carefully and honestly evaluated to allow the surgeon to plan the surgical approach, the tools and equipment that should be used, and whether or not the case can or should be performed using a minimally invasive approach at all.

PATIENT OPTIMIZATION

Patients should be medically optimized before surgery whenever possible. Anemia, diabetes, asthma, and other such comorbidities should be addressed long before going to the OR. Successful optimization often includes collaborative clearance by a primary care provider or medical subspecialist. Pre-operative hormonal optimization can also be helpful in many scenarios. For example, hormonal suppression with GnRH-agonists has been shown to reduce uterine and fibroid volume and increase pre-operative hemoglobin levels. As a result, intraoperative blood loss, OR time, and complication rates have been shown to be reduced when a pre-operative GnRH-agonist was used.[9]

PATIENT POSITIONING: WHY IS THIS IMPORTANT?

Once in the OR, the next important step in ensuring a safe surgery is properly positioning the patient under anesthesia to prevent nerve injury. Post-operative neuropathies are estimated to occur in 1.8% to 1.9% of vaginal and other major pelvic surgeries, respectively.[10,11] They can be caused by improper patient positioning, particularly in lengthy operations, poorly positioned stirrups, inadequate padding, and direct compression of peripheral nerves. Direct nerve injury can also occur during the improper closure of lower lateral trocar sites in laparoscopic surgery.[12] To understand and prevent iatrogenic neurologic injury, knowledge of anatomy, including the location and course of the most commonly injured nerves along with their relationship to nearby bony structures and other important landmarks is of paramount importance. In this way, surgeons can understand how nerves become compressed, stretched, and disrupted during the operation, leading to both sensory and motor neuropathies.[13,14]

The incidence of malposition-related injuries in gynecologic laparoscopy is estimated at between 0.02% and 0.16% in the upper limbs and between 1.5% and 1.8% in the lower limbs and at less than 1% in robotic-assisted surgeries. The exact incidence is not well known because of underreporting and self-resolution of most injuries because the overwhelming majority will recover over time unless overtly transected without repair. Patient-specific factors that may put them at higher risk for iatrogenic nerve injury include very high or very low BMI, age greater than 60 years, a history of smoking or alcohol intake, and hypovolemia, hypotension, electrolyte imbalance, or malnutrition at the time of surgery.[14] Nerve injury sites most commonly encountered during minimally invasive gynecologic surgery include the brachial plexus, ulnar, femoral, common peroneal, iliohypogastric, and ilioinguinal nerves.

Previous studies have demonstrated an increased frequency of nerve injuries associated with increased surgical time spent in lithotomy position. One study showed a 100-fold increase in likelihood of injury with each additional hour in lithotomy position.[15] Surgeries over 2 hours long were previously associated with a significantly increased risk of nerve injury.[16] However, more recent studies did not find strong evidence suggesting increased neuropathy with increased operative time.[17–19] Likely mechanisms of injury, and so too the corresponding preventive measures, center on patient positioning in low dorsal lithotomy and known anatomic relationships.[13,14]

Avoiding the Post-operative Neuropathy: Optimal Positioning and Padding

To prevent compression injuries of the common peroneal and ulnar nerves, care must be taken in positioning of the legs in stirrups or tucking the arms against the OR table. Extra padding can be placed to provide a cushion to protect the nerves where they run superficially and are at greatest risk. Compression of the femoral nerve where it runs under the inguinal ligament, as well as the lateral femoral cutaneous nerve as it courses over the iliacus, can both occur with excessive hip flexion greater than 80° to 90°, or extreme abduction and external rotation while in the lithotomy position, or even if the patient's inner thigh is leaned on excessively during surgery.[13] In procedures in which the arms are not tucked against the OR table, stretch injuries can occur at the brachial plexus when the arms are improperly positioned on arm boards and abducted greater than 90° for long periods of time.

Trendelenburg Without the Slide

There are numerous devices aimed at preventing patient displacement on the OR table during steep Trendelenburg while also reducing pressure and minimizing the risk of neuropathy. The rate of neuropathy is low overall, with a 0.16% incidence across 5 studies including 1923 patients in a recent systematic review. However, it is remains impossible to make clear recommendations on ideal positioning techniques or devices because of the lack of head-to-head studies and the heterogeneity of available studies. Large, multi-center trials comparing these techniques, designed to measure both patient displacement and neuropathy, are needed.[18]

Shoulder braces are available to prevent cephalad slide with steep Trendelenburg but can cause compression and stretch injuries. Placement of the braces too far medially, close to the patient's neck, can cause injury as the nerves are compressed against the first rib. Placement too far laterally can cause stretch injury as gravity pulls the patient cephalad in Trendelenburg. When used, shoulder braces should be placed directly over the acromioclavicular joint; however, even this positioning does not completely prevent the risk of injury.[13] As a result, some advocate for avoiding the use of shoulder braces altogether.[14] However, recent studies have shown that shoulder braces can be safely used, in combination with a beanbag system with or without egg crate foam, to effectively prevent patient slide without an increased risk of neurologic injury.[15,20] Beanbags, egg crate, or foam mattress pads can also be used without shoulder braces to prevent sliding during surgery, although they are less effective at preventing sliding. A recent meta-analysis found that the use of the beanbag system with shoulder supports/braces was superior to memory foam with a chest strap or gel pads. Gel pads and memory foam with chest straps were comparable with each other in preventing patient slide. No difference was seen in comparative rates of neuropathy regardless of device used.[18]

Regardless of the devices used, surgeons must continue to focus on proper positioning with attention to padding of all pressure points with care not to hyper-flex, over-rotate, or over-abduct the limbs (**Fig. 1**). Using only the minimum amount of Trendelenburg required for adequate visualization is also important. Many surgeries can be performed efficiently without the use of very steep Trendelenburg.[21]

Apart from patient positioning-related nerve injuries, direct injuries of the ilioinguinal and iliohypogastric nerves can occur during abdominal trocar entry in the lower

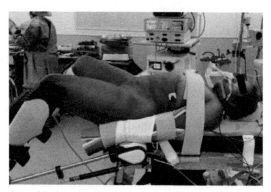

Fig. 1. Appropriately padded and positioned patient in low dorsal lithotomy.

quadrants. Careful placement of ports away from the course of the nerves is most important in preventing direct injury. Nerves can also be entrapped and compressed during the closure of fascial defects. The use of radial-dilating trocars or those whose defects do not need to be closed and avoiding very tight closures can also help.[12]

LAPAROSCOPIC ENTRY: WHAT'S THE BIG DEAL ABOUT GAINING PERITONEAL ACCESS?

Most complications occur during abdominal entry; the most dangerous part of a laparoscopic procedure. Complications can be minor, including insufflation of the subcutaneous tissue leading to subcutaneous emphysema and extra-peritoneal insufflation and post-operative infection. However, they can also be major and life threatening, including injury to major blood vessels or viscera. In a 2000 study of laparoscopic surgery malpractice claims, trocars were associated with injury more than any other laparoscopic device, making up 31% of claims. Veress needles made up 8% of claims.[22] From January 1, 1997, to June 30, 2002, the US Food and Drug Administration's Manufacturer and User Facility Device Experience database received 1353 reports of nonfatal trocar-related injuries and 46 reports on 31 separate fatal trocar-related injuries. A total of 74% of the deaths were associated with blood loss from vascular injuries, with most specified cases resulting from injury to major vessels, including the aorta, the iliac artery/vein, and the vena cava. The remaining cases involved bowel injury or injury to the stomach or gastric vessels and 1 case of peritonitis. Interestingly, 10% of these cases were gynecologic in nature.[23]

Peritoneal Access Techniques

A variety of laparoscopic trocars have been developed in the hopes of minimizing trocar injury at entry (**Fig. 2**). Many different techniques have also been developed to assist in entry and minimize risk. A 2015 Cochrane review including 26 randomized controlled trials with 3 multi-arm trials evaluated 13 laparoscopic entry techniques and found no evidence of advantage using any single instrument or technique for preventing major vascular or visceral complications. The open-entry (Hasson) technique is associated with a lower risk of failed entry than the other techniques, but with no difference in injury to viscera or vasculature. For closed techniques, there was a lower risk of failed entry and vascular injury when direct trocar entry was used compared with Veress needle entry. Overall, when comparing direct optical entry, Veress needle, radially expanding trocars (STEP trocars), direct entry without prior insufflation and open-entry techniques, there was insufficient evidence to recommend one technique over another.[24]

However, because complications remain rare, most trials comparing techniques are inadequately powered to detect statistically significant differences. Most studies included in the Cochrane review were of low or very low quality. Although the review concludes that there is insufficient evidence to recommend one laparoscopic entry technique over another, this does not mean that all techniques are equally safe hence more research is necessary. In 2016, the International Society for Gynecologic Endoscopy convened a taskforce on abdominal entry through which members analyzed existing research, literature reviews, existing international and national guidelines, and expert opinion, and presented a comprehensive collection of practical guidelines on safe laparoscopic entry.[25]

Open (Hasson) versus closed entry technique

The International Society for Gynecologic Endoscopy taskforce noted that the Hasson technique for obtaining primary trocar placement is associated with a reduced rate of

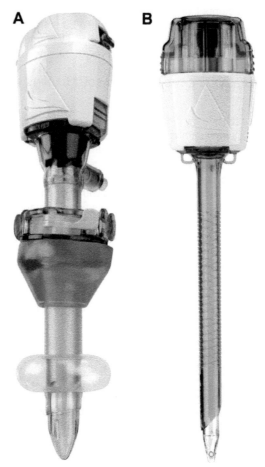

Fig. 2. (*A*) Kii Balloon Blunt Tip and (*B*) Kii Fios Z-Thread. (*Courtesy of* Applied Medical, Rancho Santa Margarita, CA.)

failed entry without significant difference in visceral or vascular injury sites. In closed techniques, a urinary catheter and nasogastric/orogastric tube should be placed before entry to help decompress viscera and decrease the risk of injury. Patients should also be horizontal during entry because Trendelenburg positioning alters the location of critical internal anatomy and increases the risk of injury. Care should be taken to identify omental and bowel adhesions or other abnormalities that can still complicate an open entry.[26]

Closed entry (Veress needle) technique
Initial insufflation with a Veress needle can be used to facilitate primary trocar placement. Standard safety precautions should be used for initial skin incision. Care should be taken not to stab right through the abdominal wall with pointed scalpel blades, particularly in very thin or pediatric patients. Grasping and elevating the lower anterior abdominal wall while placing a Veress needle at the umbilicus has not been shown to reduce the risk of injury. On the contrary, it has been associated with a significantly higher rate of failed entry so this step is not recommended. The angle of the Veress

needle during insertion should be adjusted based on the patient's BMI and the resulting change in distance between the umbilicus and the aortic bifurcation. The needle should be angled at 45° in non-obese women and 90° in morbidly obese women.

When using the umbilicus for entry, the incision should be made at the deepest point of the umbilical pit where the abdominal wall is the thinnest, independent of the patient's BMI. With umbilical entry, surgeons must also take into consideration the significant caudal displacement of the umbilicus in patients with a large pannus, or patients with history of umbilical hernia with or without repair or history of an abdominoplasty, in whom the umbilicus has been artificially moved and re-implanted thereby altering the original presumed landmarks.

Various alternative insertion sites can be used depending on the patient's medical or surgical history or to accommodate large and obstructing pathology. Adhesions are common in patients with a history of prior abdominal or pelvic surgery. Of these, intestinal adhesions are most often found in the peri-umbilical area. The rate of occurrence of bowel adhesions increases with the number of abdominal surgeries and is worse with a history of midline incisions.[27] Imaging with MRI or transabdominal ultrasound using the slide test[28] can be useful in detecting adhesions and finding adhesion-free areas before surgery.

Left upper quadrant (Palmer's point) entry may be used when there is known umbilical pathology or strong suspicion of adhesions at the umbilicus. When there is known hepatosplenomegaly, history of gastric or pancreatic masses or previous surgeries, or other conditions making Palmer's point a potentially dangerous entry point, alternative sites should be considered. The Lee Huang point (between the umbilicus and the xiphoid process), ninth intercostal space, uterine fundus, and posterior vaginal fornix have all been used and described in the literature as alternate sites for obtaining peritoneal access.[29]

After placement of the Veress needle, correct placement can be verified using a variety of tests including the saline hanging-drop and negative pressure tests. Low intra-abdominal pressures (<10 mm Hg) provide the most reliable confirmation.[29] It is important to note that the risk of injury with Veress needle insertion increases significantly with additional number of placement attempts, and reaches 44% to 74% for 3 and 85% to 100% for 4 or more attempts. It is therefore recommended that an alternate entry technique be used after 3 failed attempts with the Veress.[27]

Successful intra-peritoneal placement of the Veress needle and subsequent pneumoperitoneum elevates the fascia away from the organs and vessels and creates some tension at the level of the fascia for safer trocar placement. It is important to balance the negative effects of high intra-abdominal pressure, including cardiovascular stress and decreased lung compliance, with safety and visibility during the procedure. In gynecologic surgery, one must also take into account the added stress of steep Trendelenburg position. An individual patient's cardiopulmonary status and body habitus must also be taken into consideration. Ongoing communication with the anesthesia team will also be an important determinant of potential limitations. Despite the physiologic changes imposed by pneumoperitoneum, in most healthy patients, an intra-abdominal pressure of 25 mm Hg can be safely used for primary trocar insertion. The pressure can then be decreased to the usual 12 to 16 mm Hg after all trocars have been inserted.

Direct trocar insertion without prior insufflation

Directly inserting a sharp and pointed trocar at the level of the umbilicus without pneumoperitoneum avoids the risks and additional time associated with Veress needle placement. Although direct entry is associated with fewer failures and less extra-peritoneal insufflation, the intra-abdominal injuries made can be more cata-strophic given the often larger caliber of the trocar.[26] Randomized controlled trials are available but none are powered to detect differences in major complications, hence there is insufficient evidence to recommend this method over other methods.[27]

Innovations in trocar technology

Radially expanding trocars have been available since the early 1990s and have shown reduced rates of entry failure and extra-peritoneal insufflation, but there is no evidence of significant differences in vascular, visceral, or solid organ injuries. Optical trocars allow for continuous visualization of the layers of the abdominal wall as the trocar passes through them. Optical threaded trocars, which the surgeon places by screwing the device in at the incision while viewing the progress through the abdominal wall, allows for a more controlled entry than the traditional push-through trocars. The cannula's threads also work to tent the tissue layers upward during placement. Studies have shown a reduced risk of injury during entry using these ports.[29]

SUMMARY

Once an appropriately indicated procedure is identified in a medically optimized patient, surgery can begin. A proper fund of neuroanatomical knowledge during posi-tioning of a patient in low dorsal lithotomy minimizes the risk of sustaining a post-operative neuropathy. Similarly, familiarity with a variety of peritoneal access techniques facilitates selecting the safest and most effective abdominal entry approach. By having a well thought out strategy from start to finish, the benefits of MIS can be fully realized.

REFERENCES

1. Aarts JW, Nieboer TE, Johnson N, et al. Surgical approaches to hysterectomy for benign gynaecological disease. Cochrane Database Syst Rev 2015;(8):CD003677.
2. Colling KP, Colling KP, Glover JK, et al. Abdominal hysterectomy: reduced risk of surgical site infection associated with robotic and laparoscopic technique. Surg Infect (Larchmt) 2015;16(5):498–503.
3. Gandaglia G, Ghani KR, Sood A, et al. Effect of minimally invasive surgery on the risk for surgical site infections: results from the National Surgical Quality Improve-ment Program (NSQIP) database. JAMA Surg 2014;149(10):1039–44.
4. Louie M, Strassle PD, Moulder JK, et al. Uterine weight and complications after abdominal, laparoscopic, and vaginal hysterectomy. Am J Obstet Gynecol 2018;219(5):480.e1-8.
5. Catanzarite T, Saha S, Pilecki MA, et al. Longer operative time during benign laparoscopic and robotic hysterectomy is associated with increased 30 day peri-operative complications. J Minim Invasive Gynecol 2015;22(6):1049–58.
6. Wallace SK, Fazzari MJ, Chen H, et al. Outcomes and postoperative complica-tions after hysterectomies performed for benign compared with malignant indica-tions. Obstet Gynecol 2016;128(3):467–75.
7. Suidan RS, He W, Sun CC, et al. Impact of body mass index and operative approach on surgical morbidity and costs in women with endometrial carcinoma and hyperplasia. Gynecol Oncol 2017;145(1):55–60.
8. Committee on Gynecologic Practice. Committee Opinion No 701: choosing the route of hysterectomy for benign disease. Obstet Gynecol 2017;129:e155-9.

9. Lethaby A, Puscasiu L, Vollenhoven B. Preoperative medical therapy before surgery for uterine fibroids. Cochrane Database Syst Rev 2017;(11):CD000547.

10. Bohrer JC, Walters MD, Park A, et al. Pelvic nerve injury following gynecologic surgery: a prospective cohort study. Am J Obstet Gynecol 2009;201: 531.

11. Cardosi RJ, Cox CS, Hoffman MS. Postoperative neuropathies after major pelvic surgery. Obstet Gynecol 2002;100:240–4.

12. Shin JH, Howard FM. Abdominal wall nerve injury during laparoscopic gynecologic surgery: incidence, risk factors, and treatment outcomes. J Minim Invasive Gynecol 2012;19:448–53.

13. Bradshaw AD, Advincula AP. Postoperative neuropathy in gynecologic surgery. Obstet Gynecol Clin North Am 2010;37:451–9.

14. Abdalmageed OS, Bedaiwy MA, Falcone T. Nerve injuries in gynecologic laparoscopy. J Minim Invasive Gynecol 2017;24(1):16–27.

15. Warner MA, Martin JT, Schroeder DR, et al. Lower extremity motor neuropathy associated with surgery performed on patients in a lithotomy position. Anesthesiology 1994;81:6–12.

16. Warner MA, Warner DO, Harper CM, et al. Lower extremity neuropathies associated with lithotomy positions. Anesthesiology 2000;93:938–42.

17. Treszezamsky AD, Fenske S, Moshier EL, et al. Neurologic injury and patient displacement in gynecologic laparoscopic surgery using a beanbag and shoulder supports. Int J Gynaecol Obstet 2018;140(1):26–30.

18. Das D, Propst K, Wechter ME, et al. Evaluation of positioning devices for optimization of outcomes in laparoscopic and robotic-assisted gynecologic surgery. J Minim Invasive Gynecol 2019;26(2):244–52.e1.

19. Klauschie J, Wechter ME, Jacob K, et al. Use of anti-skid material and patient positioning to prevent patient shifting during robotic-assisted gynecologic procedures. J Minim Invasive Gynecol 2010;17(4):504–7.

20. Farag S, Rosen L, Ascher-Walsh C. Comparison of the memory foam pad versus the bean bag with shoulder braces in preventing patient displacement during gynecologic laparoscopic surgery. J Minim Invasive Gynecol 2018; 25(1):153–7.

21. Ghomi A, Kramer C, Askari R, et al. Trendelenburg position in gynecologic robotic-assisted surgery. J Minim Invasive Gynecol 2012;19:485–9.

22. Bartholomew L, Traywick R, Quinn R, et al. Laparoscopic injury study. "Insuring the practice of quality healthcare". Rockville, MD: Physician Insurers Association of America; 2000.

23. Fuller J, Ashar BS, Carey-Corrado J. Trocar-associated injuries and fatalities: an analysis of 1399 reports to the FDA. J Minim Invasive Gynecol 2005;12(4):302–7.

24. Ahmad G, Gent D, Henderson D, et al. Laparoscopic entry techniques. Cochrane Database Syst Rev 2015;(8):CD006583.

25. Taskforce for Abdominal Entry. Principles of safe laparoscopic entry. Eur J Obstet Gynecol Reprod Biol 2016;201:179–88.

26. Siufi Neto J, Santos Siufi DF, Magrina JF. Trocar in conventional laparoscopic and robotic-assisted surgery as a major cause of iatrogenic trauma to the patient. Best Pract Res Clin Obstet Gynaecol 2016;35:13–9.

27. Okabayashi K, Ashrafian H, Zacharakis E, et al. Adhesions after abdominal surgery: a systematic review of the incidence distribution and severity. Surg Today 2014;l44(3):405–20.

28. Zinther NB, Fedder J, Friis-Andersen H. Noninvasive detection and mapping of intraabdominal adhesions: a review of the current literature. Surg Endosc 2010; 24(11):2681–6.
29. Ternamian AM, Vilos GA, Vilos AG, et al. Laparoscopic peritoneal entry with the reusable threaded visual cannula. J Minim Invasive Gynecol 2010;17(4):461–7.

Printed and bound by CPI Group (UK) Ltd, Croydon, CR0 4YY

03/10/2024

01040402-0001